Insight and ea

MY CALLING

CHRONICLES
of an
ALASKAN
HOSPICE NURSE

Esther Pepper RN, BSN, CHPN

My Calling Chronicles of an Alaskan Hospice Nurse
Copyright © 2024 by Esther Pepper RN, BSN, CHPN. All rights reserved.

The names and identifying details in the stories featured in this book have been changed to protect the privacy and confidentiality of individuals. Any resemblance to real persons, living or deceased, is purely coincidental.

Neither the publisher nor the author is engaged in rendering professional advice or services to the individual reader. The ideas, procedures and suggestions contained in this book are not intended as a substitute for consulting with your physician. All matters regarding your health require medical supervision. Neither the author nor the publisher shall be liable or responsible for any loss or damage allegedly arising from any information or suggestions in this book.

No part of this book may be used or reproduced in any manner whatsoever without written permission, except in the case of brief quotations embodied in critical articles and reviews. For more information, e-mail all inquiries to info@manhattanbookgroup.com.

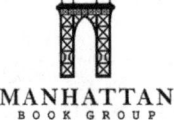

Published by Manhattan Book Group
447 Broadway 2nd Floor, #354, New York, NY 10013
(212) 634-7677 | www.manhattanbookgroup.com

Book Cover Photo credits to ET Clark
Author Photo credits to Danielle Mehler

Printed in the United States of America.
ISBN: 978-1-965340-46-2 (Paperback)
       978-1-966074-06-9 (Hardcover)

Dedicated to the called hospice nurses, to the chosen ones of the future and to every caregiver who has witnessed their loved ones crossing over.

Contents

Introduction. vii
Acknowledgments ix

A Tale of Three Men 1
I Will Decide 23
One in a Million 35
I'll Do It My Way. 41
Springtime. 47
Soaring with Eagles. 53
The Pause 59
The Ceiling is the Limit 73
Addendum 81
Till Death Us Do Part 85
Patience 97
Speed it Up 105
Cultural Diversities 113
The Doctors Role. 117
The Power of Words 125
In Shock. 129
White Out on the Snow Moon. 137

GIP: General Inpatient Level of Care	145
Terminal Agitation	151
Seismic 7.1	159
The Love of a Sister	165
The Good Samaritan	171
Gina	179
My Vet	185
Life Review	193
Excentric Exit	201
Once Upon a Storytime	207
In the Beginning	215
Darkness	219
Love is Blue	223
Travel Talk	227
Boundaries	233
Aurora	235
Conclusion	237
Resource Page	239

Introduction

The Chronicles offers insight and education for end-of-life care, including pain and symptom management on specific disease processes. The stories are for Hospice Nurses and caregivers, providing care for patients and loved ones. The Chronicles of love, endurance, faithful companionship, and pain will inspire you as you experience the stories unfold in the Alaskan setting.

The Chronicles include 25 different disease processes, remarkable caregivers, the grieving processes, the four levels of care Hospice provides, and healthy boundaries that need to be in place with patient and caregiver relationships. Practical information is shared about the disease process when one enters Hospice and the journey experienced until the patient dies. You will find beauty in seeing the elements of the physical, mental, spiritual and emotional being and how those intertwine in each patient's story. Caregivers will gain insight into symptoms associated with each disease and how to provide comfort to their family members.

Hospice Nurses often feel a calling to this type of nursing. One way or another, we were drawn into it. Most nurses don't say, "I want to deal with death and dying every day!" Over the course of one's life, you engage and meet with circumstances that compel you to learn more about this process of life that is so taboo in our Western culture. The spark in your heart for end-of-life caregiving develops over time leading you to support and grow that passion with more knowledge and purpose.

Caregivers who can care for their loved ones and participate in the process; whether in a skilled facility, assisted living home, hospital, and in the home setting; are a resource of strength and kindness to the patient when walking this journey. You are loved and appreciated by every Hospice team member!

Some stories will invoke deep emotion. Not everyone has a peaceful death. You will explore the reasons why this can happen and understand this concept more after diving into the pages ahead!

Acknowledgments

I would like to thank the following amazing people in my life!

Mary Kay, what a sweet surprise for you to offer to be my editor after the journey with your mom was completed. Thank you for your abundant generosity and friendship.

My mom, Carlene, for your thoughtful insight and helping with the Hospice Highlights. This brought back fond memories of you editing my papers during high school.

My dad, William, you are the pillar of our family. Thank you for your love.

My sister, Beth, you gave inspiration every step of the way and brought out phrases to characterize the stories, which was an extra bonus.

My lovely children, Sabella and Simon, your love and support during my convalescence was precious. I can't imagine my life without you! My heart belongs to you.

My sweet nieces, Carly and Maddison, your physical presence and care for your Aunty when I needed you most will never be forgotten.

My sister-in-law LaRae, brother David, my niece Jessica, and Aunt Kathy, your support and help last springtime was invaluable.

My family and friends, you know who you are! Your encouraging words along the way kept me going to find fruition with this project.

My hospice work family, I am so blessed to be a part of an incredible team. What a reward it is in the career of a hospice nurse to work with a group of professionals who are genuinely full of compassion and who have set a high standard for quality patient care. Your dedication over the years holds a special place in my heart. Thank you!

A TALE OF THREE MEN

This tale shares the first time during my 15 years of hospice nursing that I encountered the phenomenon of case-managing simultaneously three patients with the most amazing spouses as caregivers. Each demonstrated devotion beyond comprehension and was an intuitive caregiver. Walking alongside them through their final months' journeys allowed me to observe how each spouse uniquely encountered the grieving process. These stories inspired me to write *My Calling*: *Chronicles of an Alaskan Hospice Nurse*.

Bargaining

My first love tale is about John. John and Mary had been married for over 56 years. Alaskan stories, adventures, and places lived were shared with me on many visits. John had been walking the long goodbye with Mary for many years through her Alzheimer's diagnosis. What precipitated Mary coming on to service was a fall that needed evaluation and landed her in the hospital emergency room. Since she had experienced several falls in a short time frame, she was referred to hospice. As more practitioners observe the pattern of decline in this disease process, more precious folks are admitted to comfort care months ahead versus the last week or two of life.

John paid meticulous attention to Mary's daily routine from early morning until nighttime. Every morning, his priority was to get her dressed and up to the living room by the crackling, warm wood stove in their cabin. This became much more difficult over time as Mary required almost complete care now and couldn't help in any way.

They lived in a remote area outside of town. Added to that difficulty was the fact that they lived in a dry cabin, meaning there was no heat or indoor plumbing. Let me clarify: there was no running water, no septic, or natural gas heat. John cooked on a propane stove, and the cabin was heated by a wood stove. Up until this point, John had chopped all their wood. The container for elimination in the bathroom was coined a 'honey bucket.' I didn't ask where it was dumped. Thank goodness they at least had electricity.

John had built the house in sections and layers, as many Alaskans often do. It wasn't finished on the inside, with drywall still needed, as well as siding on the outside. There were unfinished projects throughout the cabin. The ability to navigate safely through the cabin was akin to an art form that included balance and heightened spatial awareness. It was easy to stumble if you weren't paying attention.

John ensured Mary had meals, no matter how challenging it became for her to eat. He was very patient, often taking an hour to walk her to the kitchen and feed her breakfast. Mary responded to John well in the early months of being on service. She knew her husband's tender voice and would call out when she needed him.

As digression occurred cognitively, she became weaker. The falls continued as her behavior and movement were spontaneous. There was no holding her back. On one adventure, she managed to get out the front door and down the five steps to the driveway.

Fortunately, it was late autumn and not too cold with freezing temperatures when John caught her walking feebly down the driveway toward the main road. John agreed to install a door alarm after this event, along with a simple video monitoring system to help watch her so he could do tasks in the house and outside.

We worked with John to provide the CTI (Certificate of Terminal Illness) from our medical director to the court system as he was finalizing Mary's guardianship paperwork. We also called the Medicaid social worker to explain Mary's need to get her PCA

(Personal Care Assistant) hours increased in the system. It took a few weeks to establish this increase, which allowed John to run errands and do household chores.

Living in a dry cabin in Alaska is challenging, to say the least. Along with being a full-time elderly caregiver, John had projects inside the house as well as outside. Through all the falling events, I believe Mary's angels were busy safeguarding her as no broken bones occurred. Her faith had been strong for decades, and her passion ran deep for God. It was amazing to see and hear her reading from her large print Bible, making no mistakes in her oration.

About every three weeks during the 5½ months Mary was on service, she developed a low-grade fever that would last several days and then resolve. No other signs of a urinary tract infection (UTI) or other upper respiratory symptoms were present. She would sleep more during these times and eat less, leading to progressive weight loss. The overall amount of food she ate became less consistent, with breakfast usually being the better meal of the day.

This was hard for John to watch. I encouraged him to let her rest in bed these days, but he struggled with that, too. It was important for John to keep the routine going as she would spend most of her day in the living room chair while he was doing chores in the house.

As her disease progressed, Mary's gait and ability to walk drastically declined, and guided assistance was no longer possible. She would stand but could not get her legs to move properly. John cleared space in the cabin so that the wheelchair could go from the bed to the living room chair where she spent most of her day.

As nutrition decreased, her skin deteriorated with redness on her tailbone. Doing the side-to-side tilt to offload the pressure in her recliner chair was difficult as it was very narrow. Redness started with a stage one pressure injury to the coccyx. Shortly after, she had one of her fever spells, and John allowed her to stay in bed to rest (after much coaxing from me). She was in bed for several days. I applied a foam dressing for protection as the sore had developed into a stage two pressure injury. Pillow rotation was easier in the bed because it had an air mattress.

During these days of fever, she didn't eat much or take fluids well. The reality of her decline was starting to set in with John, and he would become tearful. However, when the fever broke, she ate easier again, and this encouraged John that there would be more days with his bride. John was riding the rollercoaster of the grieving process, bargaining for any additional time he could.

John spent extensive effort getting Mary to the bathroom. Her ability to recognize when she needed to go declined, and she became completely incontinent. John was getting tired and exhausted, frankly, and it was affecting his health.

When I arrived at noon one day, John was lying in his bed next to Mary's. Fortunately, the personal care assistant (PCA) was present to tend to Mary's needs. John had been in bed for 15 hours and couldn't get up due to severe vertigo. He was pale with the look of complete exhaustion. I called his doctor, and they saw him the next day to adjust his meds.

I strongly requested that Respite needed to happen now! It was past time for him to have a break. Respite is one of the four levels of hospice care offered by Medicare. He reluctantly agreed. Mary spent four nights and five days in our contracted facility.

The first day she was there, John asked if he could visit and was worried they wouldn't know what to do if she was afraid. I assured him she would be fine and I would check in with Mary and the facility to see that things went smoothly. I asked him to stay home and rest; he complied. During this time Mary slept quite a bit, her decline continuing.

When she returned home, John had renewed energy, but it was too difficult for him to get Mary on and off the commode. I asked if we could insert the Foley catheter to help her skin condition on the tailbone as it was worsening. The pressure injury was now advancing from a stage three to an unstageable purple, dark area with a hard, raised red lump in the center that was hot to the touch.

Keeping her skin dry from urine was imperative. Previously, John had been reluctant to proceed with this step as he was concerned about infection. I told him if that occurred, we could manage the catheter with irrigation and possibly antibiotics if the symptoms were severe and causing discomfort. I explained the pros outweighed the cons at this point.

He agreed, and a Foley catheter was placed. Mary didn't seem to mind it at all. After the catheter insertion, Mary relaxed even more since she didn't have to get to the bathroom or have her briefs changed so often.

Food intake was minimal as she didn't know what to do with food placed in her mouth. I asked the family to stop feeding her as they had to clear her mouth from food left in her cheek each time. Explaining aspiration risk and what that meant in very simple terms was crucial. Not feeding loved ones with this disease is challenging to comprehend and accept for the caregiver. Thoughts of, "I'm withholding food, I'm starving them," settle in the background.

Sometimes, a nurse has to explain this on different levels and in various ways for families to fully understand. Force-feeding does not extend one's life or bring any quality when one can't swallow effectively.

I texted the three children, two of whom lived out of state, informing them of Mary's decline. They were very appreciative of the rallying call and arrived three days later. What ensued over the next 12 days was beautiful to watch. There was much bustling around the house as the kids helped Dad with projects and re-organization. Meals were cooked, and siblings bossed each other around amidst laughter and storytelling.

Mary didn't want to let go. I think she truly enjoyed listening to her family being together in such an intimate way. But, two days after the kids arrived, Mary stopped all oral intake. I applied the Scopolamine patch behind her ear to help dry up secretions in her lungs, as I could hear some wet crackles.

Twenty-four hours after the patch was applied, she started to have involuntary jerking movements in her legs. It kept increasing, so the patch was removed, and her legs settled down the next day. This is a *rare* adverse reaction of the Scopolamine patch called Anticholinergic Syndrome. Even with therapeutic dosages of Scopolamine, this reaction can include confusion, hallucinations, and restlessness[1]. Mary displayed psychomotor symptoms of restlessness and fidgeting of her legs.

---

[1] Osmosis, "Anticholinergics," https://www.osmosis.org/answers/anticholinergics.

During these last days, Mary consistently ran fevers, which were managed with Tylenol suppositories. Liquid morphine and Haldol in small doses a couple of times per day with a low-dose Fentanyl patch assisted with pain and anxiety associated with rolling and turning her in bed. Doing the wound care didn't seem to hurt Mary; it was more about rolling in bed and weight shifting. The purple-black color of the wound, which was unstageable, had opened up to a deep stage four with much drainage. It required daily wound care and packing from the nurse as two family members helped roll and turn her gently.

John was able to give her permission to go six days before she transitioned to the next realm. Mary eventually took her last breath after very low respirations, between four and eight per minute over the last 48 hours, and she was surrounded by her faithful husband and three children. Walking alongside and supporting this sweet couple during their journey was a privilege. John's loyalty and devotion to Mary were truly exquisite to witness and be a part of. John *bargained* for more time every final step in Mary's last days. He did so with love and gentleness while caring for her in their dry cabin, their home of many years.

Hospice Highlights

- Provide counsel on how to manage best each stage of decline.
- Instruct the caregiver on where to obtain additional support and how to install household devices for safety.
- Watch for caregiver's level of exhaustion and health status: initiate Respite Care.
- Observe for possible adverse reactions to new medications initiated.
- Offer support and assistance for communication with additional family members.

Source

1) Osmosis. "Anticholinergics." https://www.osmosis.org/answers/anticholinergics.

Anger and Denial

This is a hard story to tell, but one of the purposes of this book is to educate, encourage, and nurture the next generation of Hospice nurses. You won't find these lessons in your typical "pain and symptom management" Hospice manual.

The love tale of Jerry and Debbie spans many decades. They met as teenagers. This was a challenging case due to circumstances in their history and the tragedy that happened early in their marriage. The admissions nurse advised that Jerry may need special grief counseling after Debbie passed.

In my experience in this profession, I have learned that *complicated and unresolved grief* is often rooted in unforgiveness, which can produce the coping mechanism of anger[2]. This expression of anger can be displayed in various ways and to many people.

Debbie came on to service with a diagnosis of ovarian cancer with comorbidities of multiple sclerosis and dementia. There was also a history of Obsessive Compulsive Disorder (OCD) and obsessive worrying.

Around 7 pm, the sundowner's symptoms would worsen, and agitation increased through the nighttime hours. The admitting nurse indicated I was *not to say* I was the Hospice nurse or that Debbie was on hospice services. Jerry was fearful that if she knew, her agitation would worsen, and she would have crying spells.

Often, I believe that people's understanding of the dying process is that the patient has no clue what's going on in their body. I strongly disagree with this assertion. I have come to appreciate the person who knows best about what is transpiring in their own body is the PATIENT! (Even if they have Alzheimer's or cognitive deficits).

The day after admission, the social worker and I met Jerry. The family had hired a Certified Nursing Assistant (CNA), and she was also at the table. It was clear Jerry was angry in general and having

---

[2] Psychology Today, "6 Signs of Unresolved Grief," https://www.psychology-today.com/us/blog/fixing-families/i 202310/6-signs-of-unresolved-grief.

a difficult time accepting Debbie was on hospice. Even though he had signed the paperwork the previous day, he was in *denial* that this was happening.

The family stated they were past the point of being able to redirect Debbie, and offering distraction therapy was no longer working to calm her down. The medication, Seroquel, was also not effective at the current dosage. Our medical director worked with Jerry on a dosage regimen to titrate this medication.

A plan was created that I would visit three times a week and check Debbie over briefly with vital signs and assessment. Then, I would proceed to another part of the house, away from Debbie, to discuss how she was doing with Jerry. Jerry was in denial of the severity of the situation and why she was put on hospice. His focus was on the diagnosis of multiple sclerosis/dementia symptoms. She came on to service because the ovarian cancer was spreading. Her abdomen was distended, and she was experiencing intermittent bleeding vaginally.

When folks come on to Hospice, it is often recommended by the medical director to pare down the medication list from their 20-plus pills a day to only the essentials for pain and symptom management. As nutritional intake lessens, mobility declines and alertness reduces. Metabolically, it is very difficult to process medications properly. Reducing her medication list was not something that Jerry wanted to do. He stated, "If she doesn't have her MS meds, it will get worse, and she won't be able to walk anymore or move. All of these meds are keeping her going."

He had a hard time understanding that hospice would not pay for medications not related to the terminal diagnosis, but his insurance supplemental card would cover it. After being on the receiving end of much verbal anger, I asked Jerry if he really wanted our services to help Debbie, as she was declining. I was ready to walk out the door. I stated, "I don't have to be here if you don't want our help." He calmed down and apologized.

I called the insurance company to clarify coverage so Jerry could understand. They assured Jerry that the "other" meds would be covered 100% and would be delivered every three months. He also had no deductible for these prescriptions. I explained that the pain and agitation meds would be covered by the hospice Medicare benefit and filled locally by our pharmacy.

Over the next few weeks, we worked with the medical director, advising on the Seroquel dosage and liquid Ativan to help with nighttime behaviors. We saw only minor improvements, and Debbie continued to decline. Stopping the daily aspirin helped with the intermittent vaginal bleeding. Her abdomen remained distended with the Metastasis process. As needed, Tylenol helped with low-grade fevers. Overall, Debbie did not have any pain issues.

Food intake was important for Jerry to oversee, and she continued to eat most of her meals. But eventually, that started to decrease and her sleep increased with naps during the day. I showed Jerry excerpts from the book *Gone From My Sight*, how Debbie's symptoms indicated she only had a few weeks rather than months left. He was tearful. It was hard for Jerry to hear that less food intake would occur and that it was ok.

We got to a place in the nurse-caregiver relationship where the visits were methodical. I would teach, and Jerry would listen. One day, when he was tearful, I offered a supportive hug, and he readily accepted. This became our ritual at the end of every visit. I believe Jerry appreciated the compassionate gesture.

I was on call the weekend the call came in. This was a night I will never forget, and it is forever embedded in my hippocampus! This Alaskan winter was proving to be extra special indeed, with a high windstorm (over 100 mph) and extensive power outages. You know, the kind of storm the *"lower 48"* assigns special names to. In Alaska, we buck up and deal with it… no need to assign a name to help everyone cope during the drama.

My first obstacle to conquer was to clear a downed birch tree in the patient's subdivision at midnight. Fortunately, it was a small tree, and most of the branches had already broken off. I stumbled out of my car into a 3-foot snowdrift, bundled in multiple layers and a face mask with a headlamp on. I only picked up the branches that I had to and feebly threw them off into the ditch.

I'm sure only a minute had passed, but I was beginning to feel like a statue. My hands were not cooperating with me, already stiff from the cold. The temperature with wind chill was negative 40 degrees

Fahrenheit. It was so hard to breathe through the mask. I don't know how North Slope workers do this for weeks at a time.

Next, I picked up the tree, guessing it weighed around 80 pounds or so, and shoved it off into the ditch, battling the bitter wind. I moved back to my car as quickly as possible, as I couldn't feel my fingers anymore, even with double gloves on. My eyes were practically frozen shut, eyelashes glazed with crystals. It's amazing what our bodies can do when the adrenaline is flowing!

I finally arrived at Debbie's house. My next complication to tackle was trying to stay upright while rooting around in my bin of supplies in my trunk: chux, wipes, and the Macey catheter, just in case. It felt like five minutes had passed as I collected everything while trying to stay upright in the vortex of churning wind.

Jerry greeted me at the door with a look of complete exasperation. He wasn't the only one! I quickly took off all my gear as Jerry led me to the bathroom. Debbie had thrown up a copious amount of undigested food and was on the floor, hunched over next to the bathtub. Jerry couldn't get her up. She was listless and not responding. It was clear she had experienced a neurological event. She was also running a high fever.

We cleaned her up as best we could quickly and both of us lifted her to the wheelchair and got her into bed. Debbie was still not responding to any stimulation. Her lungs had rhonchi sounds throughout, meaning she had aspirated this meal and possibly also the prior day's meals.

I called the medical director to report the findings. I wrote orders for scheduled Ativan to keep her symptoms under control. I put him on speakerphone because I needed backup! I believe Jerry needed to understand from the authority of the doctor what measures to implement. He explained the importance of scheduled comfort medications to keep Debbie's symptoms under control. It was imperative that Jerry heard the instructions directly from the doctor as his coping mechanism still had underlying denial and anger.

Did I forget to mention we were operating in the dark? Candles and headlamps guided me during this crisis call, while kerosene heat kept the house warm. Fortunately, Debbie was not using continual oxygen as the backup tanks only lasted a few hours without electricity.

Debbie was placed on daily visits as it was clear she was in her last days. Family members were supportive, and the CNA provided personal care and help.

Several days into her last week, we started low-dose morphine to help alleviate discomfort while doing all her care in the bed. The Macy catheter for rectal administration provided much ease in medication administration, especially with her swallowing difficulty and aspiration risk. This gave Jerry some control in the process, but he was losing all control, with Debbie slowly slipping away.

After three days, she was ready for a low-dose Fentanyl patch, which Jerry applied in the afternoon. I explained to him how long it took to start working. At the five-hour mark, he noticed her respirations increasing, so he removed the patch, gave morphine and Ativan, and her breathing immediately calmed down. He told the medical director he had removed it. The doctor said that was ok even though he hadn't seen side effects of an increase in respiratory pattern with Fentanyl before. He supported continued as-needed morphine and scheduled lorazepam.

The next day, when I checked in, I mentioned that I was also surprised to hear that Fentanyl caused this reaction. Once again, I was on the receiving end of some anger. It was clear that placing blame on medication and someone else versus facing the reality that his partner was dying was how he chose to process his grief. This is how some people cope. *Denial, Anger.*

The next day, I was informed that Jerry had requested a different nurse after I had made 12 visits over the previous month. His family member apologized. "He doesn't like being told what to do." Debbie died the next day surrounded by her family. I think she did find peace in the end. Jerry showed much devotion and love to his bride of over 50 years.

Looking back, I believe Debbie suffered from *Terminal Restlessness* from the day we admitted her. She was on service for just over 4 weeks (usually, terminal restlessness is seen 2 to 3 weeks before passing). Her symptoms of agitation, restlessness, and difficulty sleeping at night were severe from the beginning. This was more than just sundowner's symptoms with dementia associated with the MS.

The trauma experienced early on in their life involved the sudden and tragic loss of their child, for which Debbie blamed herself. Not being able to forgive herself led to a complicated situation at the end of her life, as the agitation was inconsolable. Medications can only do so much to help in the transitioning labor pains of the physical body as it dies. Hospice pioneer, Barbara Karnes, has explained this well: *People die in the manner of how they lived.*

As hospice case managers, you must acknowledge the role grief plays with the patient and their significant other. It is unique to the individual, and recognizing complicated grief is imperative to establish healthy boundaries as a caregiver.

Yes, every once in a while, you will get "let go" as their nurse. It is okay. Make time to process this with your supervisor and your team.

The entire hospice team is needed to deliver the best care possible to the patient and family. When every member, from social worker to chaplain to CNA, is allowed to participate in helping the patient and family, it can truly make a difference. Interestingly, three months after Debbie passed, Jerry reached out to our chaplain, and he began processing his grief with one-on-one support.

Hospice Highlights

- Dealing with denial and an angry spouse or family member requires much patience and great effort to educate the reality of the end-of-life situation.
- Expect possible resistance to change in new treatment protocols compared to previous ones thought to be the best.
- In difficult situations, get backup. Put the phone on speaker or bring in another medical professional to help allay the family's fears and give further assurance to a problematic situation.
- Learn the elements of Complicated Grief: Do not be surprised that former trauma experienced in a person's life can greatly affect the dying process. Forgiveness of oneself and others is imperative for a more peaceful transition.
- If you find yourself the object of anger and are dismissed from the case, process it with your supervisor or team. Grief and the inability to control life seek an outlet. Take time to heal.

Source

2) *Psychology Today*. "6 Signs of Unresolved Grief." https://www.psychologytoday.com/us/blog/fixing-families/202310/6-signs-of-unresolved-grief.

Humor

My final love tale is of Keith and Heather. Heather came on to service with the diagnosis of Amyotrophic Lateral Sclerosis. She had been reliant upon a Trilogy ventilator for respiratory support for the previous seven months. She had no use of her arms/hands but could stand with strong support.

From the beginning of my visits with Heather, Keith was a part of every visit and attentive to all the details. It was refreshing to see that humor was an integral part of the coping strategy for this sweet couple of 36 years. The banter between this couple kept me on my toes!

We all know that humor can help cope with stress, and the repartee shared was genuinely reciprocal. At first it did take me off guard. It is rare to see coping via humor in our line of work. After all, we learned from Elizabeth Kubler Ross, that the five stages of grief are: denial, anger, bargaining, depression, and acceptance. Where, pray tell, is humor in this lineup?

Humor wasn't just a method of coping; it played a strong role in Keith's grieving process. Well, indeed, I learned from Heather and Keith. They taught this nurse, with a dry sense of humor and a straightforward type of communicator, that it is okay to accept laughter! I learned to go with their flow, time, and space.

Establishing confidence and trust is vitally important early on in the nurse-to-patient and caregiver relationship. When I started with Heather, it was once-a-week nursing visits. I could sense they wanted privacy and not too much invasion.

Heather's symptoms were mild, with occasional coughing after eating, and weight loss was present. That changed about one month later when the coughing spells increased. Keith would have to use the "cough assist machine" on Heather's lungs to help clear the wet cough following drinking or eating. After the second severe occurrence, I encouraged Keith to give her low-dose morphine drops under the tongue. This helps respiratory muscles relax after the event, and she would recover more easily.

Keith was very much in control of managing her care. However, I asked if I could increase nursing visits to two times a week as changes were happening. Heather weighed about 75 pounds. Her skin was at risk of breakdown, starting to get red on her back, and it needed to be protected.

My medical director prepared me that aspiration pneumonia would most likely be how Heather would pass. Since she was dependent on the ventilator for breathing support, the inability to swallow effectively was the next symptom to appear. I discussed with Heather what aspiration pneumonia can be like with high fevers and severe coughing and told her that appropriate medications can help alleviate her suffering. She listened intently but was not ready to *give up* eating and taking in nutrition to sustain life.

Keith told me in our outside chats that Heather intensely believed that God was going to heal her from ALS, and she had kept this belief going ever since she was diagnosed. After all, she did beat colon cancer 16 years prior. Over the following weeks, there were discussions outside on the porch with Keith about the need for nutrition. He would lightheartedly say, "If she stops eating, it's like killing her!"

I took the time to explain that not eating as the body is preparing to take flight is a normal part of any end-stage disease process. Keith listened intently. Heather's body displayed visible signs that she was losing weight no matter how many calories she was consuming. Her skin condition directly reflected this, turning red on the bony prominences. This required the application of padded foam dressings to help prevent pressure injuries.

Keith also had questions about Heather coming off the ventilator and if that meant it was like committing suicide. These are valid questions that spouses and caregivers ask. Medical providers often tell families if they don't go on a ventilator, they will die, or if they don't have a feeding tube placed, they will starve to death. I explained that being on an artificial means of respiratory support to sustain life is not a natural process at the end of life.

The ventilator was keeping her respiratory system going in an artificial way. Pushing oneself to eat and drink when the body is rejecting it is going against what your body is telling you it can handle. Most likely, Heather would pass due to aspiration because of her desire to keep eating and drinking even when her body was vividly telling her it couldn't tolerate this with the coughing spells.

Keith had been her advocate and supported her through the caregiving process with the utmost devotion for several years. A powerful realization of understanding of disease progression and acceptance came to Keith when he made the statement: "It's time for her to move on; it's time for us to move on." He must have been grieving in his heart and mind for quite some time and came to this place of acceptance.

This statement surprised me because of his positive attitude and coping with the daily routine through humor. I was beginning to see his resolve as he was grieving the loss of his bride.

I think Keith had been mourning the loss of Heather for several years as the quality of life they once had together was gone. The adventures they experienced in the Alaskan wilderness of flying, fishing, snow machining, boating, traveling the world and partnering in life had dissipated. Keith told me it had been over a year since Heather was able to go out to their cabin they had built together in the woods. It was only accessible by plane in the summer or snowmachine in winter.

After hearing the description of the 'cabin,' I told Keith, "This is not a cabin but rather a two-story house!" I was flabbergasted and asked how on earth he was able to transport her to the remote location of 80 miles through challenging terrain? He said, "It was simple. I just fastened her securely with straps to the back of the snowmachine. She would sit right behind me. This kept her upright and safe. Then I would carry her into the cabin where we had a wheelchair."

Keith was ready to let Heather transition to the next realm, and he understood that physical healing would not come in this earthly sphere but in the spiritual realm. Anticipatory grieving is a powerful experience exclusive to every individual. Many years ago, Keith had a feeling deep inside that Heather would never live to see old age after her cancer diagnosis.

Recognizing this is very important for the hospice nurse to deliver thorough and encompassing care. Nevertheless, was Heather ready to let go?

After a night of Heather gasping for air and her lips turning blue, Keith put the Trilogy ventilator on its highest setting and gave several rounds of morphine. He was discernably shaken the next morning and exhausted. I approached and asked if our nurse practitioner could meet with them to discuss the disease process and answer their questions from her perspective and knowledge. They agreed to her visit.

After the NP's visit, Heather understood better and agreed it was time to come off the ventilator. Heather did not want to see Keith suffer more. Coming off the ventilator would avoid aspiration pneumonia and the high fevers and labored respiratory distress that would ensue. We set a time for my next visit to spend the day with her for this process.

After much discussion between Heather and Keith, she decided she needed one more week before her transition. She wanted to say goodbye to her brother, son, and granddaughter and see her friends once more.

One week before her transitioning day, I explained how we could prepare and be ready. I would come out the day before and give an enema to clear her lower GI tract in preparation for the Macey catheter insertion. This would allow me to give the liquid meds of morphine and Ativan with greater viability than orally since her aspiration risk was so great.

I would spend the day with her in a "Continuous Care Session." This is one of four levels of care offered with the hospice benefit. An explanation was given for medications that would keep her comfortable. Keith would apply the 25 mcg Fentanyl patch to her skin at 6 am that morning, and I would arrive at 11:30. This would be adequate time for proper absorption of the Fentanyl. Our medical director wrote for hourly medication administration of morphine and Ativan to keep her comfortable for breathing support, symptoms, and pain if that would occur.

As hospice nurses, it is wonderful to engage with the spiritual aspect of our patients; it doesn't always have to be the chaplain, priest, rabbi, or their spiritual provider. We were taught in nursing school this element is part of who we are and part of the "nursing process." I asked permission if I could pray with Heather and Keith, and they agreed.

Embracing one's faith in their journey is a beautiful display of empathy and kindness. It is an honor to engage in this practice with our patients. This allows surrender to the next dominion, with peace, as their life has found fruition on this physical earth. One thing specifically Heather told me that she couldn't wait to do *was to give Jesus a hug!*

On her transition day, I asked specific questions, allowing Heather to make some choices, such as: did she want me in the room the whole time with her? Or did she want me to periodically check in on her and give her some space? Did she want music playing during this time?

She knew what she wanted. Her musical preferences were unbeknownst to me, so I had prepared some selections of soft, gentle background music on my phone. I found out her only favorite was techno-pop music. That lasted about 10 minutes as the electronic dance rhythm was not a soothing background.

I was privileged to have her personal care assistant with me that day for the process and to help with her care. That truly was a blessing as there was a bond and trust with her.

I arrived at 11:30, and Keith tenderly transferred her into the hospital bed via the wheelchair. He had placed the Fentanyl patch early that morning. I applied the Scopolamine patch but didn't anticipate heavy secretions as she would most likely pass today.

After insertion of the Macey catheter, I gave morphine and Ativan. I gave her a couple of rounds to help her relax, and one hour later, the ventilator was removed. Keith spent time with her and gave her space as well. She was still alert and wanted to talk to Keith. After a while, I asked Keith to give her some time alone to help her relax more.

Keith told me later that Heather told him, "Don't delete anything from my phone… I might be back!" The humor was present even in their last words.

The background was quiet in the room, and Nicole and I checked in on her every 30 minutes at first. It took about two hours for her to drift into a deep sleep. Heather's oxygen saturation levels slowly dropped over the next several hours; eventually, saturation levels maintained at

30% for three hours. Her feet and legs started to cool and medication was given hourly to help her breathing stay comfortable.

The beauty of these continuous care sessions is that they allow hospice to support the family in a very comprehensive way during the final hours of their loved one's life. Keith was able to have his time and space when he needed it, and then he could spend moments with Heather when he was ready.

During her last 10 minutes, Heather's breathing became very shallow and sporadic, with long pauses. Her oxygen saturation readings declined to 20% and then 10%. I encouraged her that it was okay to let go and that soon, she would be *giving Jesus a hug*. I called Keith into the room to hold her once more. About 7½ hours after being removed from the Trilogy ventilator, Heather's death was one of the most peaceful crossings I have ever witnessed in my career.

She took her last breath while Keith embraced her lovingly. The peace that enveloped the room was indescribable. Heather's soul took flight into her next adventure in the spiritual realm. I could see Heather surrounded by beautiful white-capped mountains and majestic trees in the presence of her Creator, with a smile that exuded her soul. I gently removed her wedding band and placed it in Keith's hands per his request.

My Tale of Three Men has taught me something powerful about caring for my hospice patients. Grief displays itself through many platforms. It's not always the way we've been traditionally taught. With our knowledge and experience, we must consider all the variable factors and coping mechanisms caregivers will demonstrate.

It is essential to provide a safe environment, establish trust, and embrace what they are going through. Initiating healthy boundaries is critical to delivering the best nursing care possible to meet our patients' needs. This will promote a gentle transition. Serving our patients and families to enable a peaceful crossing over to the next realm should be the mission of the hospice team. As a hospice nurse, you have to be flexible and adapt to the circumstances unique to each case.

Hospice Highlights

- Be sensitive to a couple or person's need for privacy.
- Be alert to families' concerns and have a ready explanation of the physical body's decline and discuss any treatment that can cause more stress that it cannot handle anymore or the adverse reactions that would be the result.
- Understand what anticipatory grief is and how to deal with it.
- Respect a patient's faith and belief in God's intervention. Never diminish hope, but deal with the realities that are happening daily with symptom management.
- Participate in spiritual support & prayer if allowed and if you are comfortable doing so.
- Discuss a patient's options to be alone during transition: listen to favorite music, have family members near, etc. Give choices.
- Engage with the display of humor caregivers may demonstrate.

I WILL DECIDE

Visceral, Neuropathic, Psychogenic, and Somatic Pain

My first meeting with Celeste was planned for 12:00 so her caregiver could be present. I could tell she was a planner, organizer, and very detail-oriented person with that first phone call. Celeste was 62 years old with a hospice diagnosis of colon cancer with metastasis to the lymphatic system, retroperitoneum, and peritoneum. She also had secondary cancer of the bladder and metastasis to the bone. Chemotherapy-induced polyneuropathy, constipation, anxiety, depression, nausea, and vomiting were on the co-morbidity list.

She had finished all the chemotherapy and palliative radiation that the Oncologist had recommended. She was now ready to focus on pain and symptom management for however long she had left to live. Celeste embraced alternative therapy with herbal treatments and medications.

I felt this was going to be challenging with pain and symptom management as there was extensive metastasis, not just one cancer but also a secondary. She also suffered from anxiety and depression. When I first walked into Celeste's home, her auburn hair was high up in a ponytail and she sported a fun house dress as she wrestled her dogs away from the door to let me inside. These two very large and energetic labs were her babies. After greeting me, she put them outside in their fenced yard.

She introduced me to her primary caregiver, Sally. Sally told me the hours of the day she would help Celeste. I arranged my visits for after Sally's shift to try and spread out the coverage until Jacob, her husband, got home from work. Celeste told me her family was close and very caring, and she was also very well supported by the LDS Church, and the sisters would visit several times a week to help with household chores and provide companionship.

One time, I sat down next to Celeste on the couch, and she quickly informed me that I was sitting too close to her and that she needed space. I apologized, recognized her boundary, and sat on the floor next to her. Celeste was petite and weighed 115 pounds. She had the appearance of protein calorie malnutrition as the cancer was taking over her body. Her abdomen presented like that of a woman who was six months pregnant. It was firm, round, and very distended. This was the second time in my career that I had seen this large of a tumor in the abdomen with edema.

Celeste wanted to tell me her story from the very beginning before she was diagnosed with colon cancer. One year prior to her diagnosis, she began administering enemas, usually several daily, to be able to have a bowel movement. She didn't think anything of this at the time. When they found cancer a few months later, it had already progressed with metastasis, and it was aggressive.

In private, Celeste let me know her husband believed hospice's mantra was to push more narcotics and that she would become dependent on them. What I picked up after several conversations was that Celeste thought her husband believed *she* was taking too many pain and anxiety medications. The discussion ensued that she was already physically dependent on the narcotics because of the cancer pain. Differentiating between dependency for true need versus psychological dependence would be in the upcoming conversations with Jacob.

We also began the conversation of describing the pain to give our medical director a better picture so we could get her pain numbers down to a more acceptable level. Celeste liked this idea!

We focused on the location of the cancer tumors, the nature, quality, intensity, and description of the pain to fine-tune her pain management regimen. She had been on a Fentanyl patch and oxycodone for several months now, and she couldn't get her pain number down below a 4/10. When we admitted Celeste, the Fentanyl patch was at 125 mcg, and she would take 30 mg of oxycodone for breakthrough pain three to four times a day.

Each adjective that Celeste gave regarding her pain fell into every category, including Visceral, Somatic, Neuropathic, and Psychogenic. She used the words "deep squeeze, cramping, sharp, gnawing, numbness, and tingling." Anxiety and depression played a big role in how her coping manifested. She had tendencies towards OCD behavior as well.

When I met with Jacob the next day, we discussed the plan of care moving forward, as Celeste's pain was not well controlled. We reviewed symptoms from the book *Gone From My Sight*, talked about pain management, and changing the long-acting medication to methadone to target neuropathy and somatic pain. I asked Jacob to install a baby gate at the top of the steps as a safety measure to avoid falls. He did so right away.

Jacob was in agreement with the plan to switch to methadone for more targeted pain control. He understood Celeste's need for pain medicine. He was concerned she would be too sedate at times if she had too many breakthrough tablets, so he would help her keep track by putting five breakthrough meds per day in a zip-lock bag and labeled it for the day.

When I mentioned to Celeste that methadone would be an excellent medication to target her neuropathy and somatic pain, she was not agreeable to starting it right away. She worried that it was too strong of a pain medicine.

In the long run, it comes down to developing trust with your patient. Celeste had to get to know me, learn how I handled her concerns, and see if I truly understood the nature of her pain and how I would interact and get orders from the medical director. He agreed to increase the Fentanyl patch to 150 mcg for now. Celeste averaged five breakthroughs per day of oxycodone 30 mg each dose. She also needed 1 mg of Ativan at night to help her sleep.

I decided to take a shortcut to get to Celeste on my next routine visit. It was a beautiful day in November, with blue skies displaying the sun after a fresh snowfall the previous night. I wanted to soak in the farmland views next to the Hatcher Pass mountains laced with pristine white snow.

Whether driving through the mountains or around farmlands, the invigorating scenery proved to be quite therapeutic between visits. This helped with processing after being with my patient before going on to the next visit. I have learned it is important to take time throughout the day to ground my thoughts and emotions after working with each patient, even if it is just for a few minutes.

I was simply just following GPS! It clearly pointed to the route of a road that went alongside a hay farm. The road even had a *name*! It would save me six miles on my trip, and I like to be on time for visits, if not a little early. Well, that was the last time I trusted new GPS routes.

It was the second snowfall of winter, and the road appeared passable at first glance. About 200 feet in, I started to sink slowly and then into deep ruts. My downsized car proved to lack the strength needed to break free. This should have been a warning for upcoming events.

I called a tow truck, which had an estimated wait time of one hour. Then a Jeep with 4-wheel drive appeared out of nowhere, zipping along the shortcut, having fun 4x4ing in the muck. He pulled up in front of me and, of course, had a few laughs at my expense. He quickly pulled me out, and I was on my way.

I was late for my visit, but Celeste quickly forgave me when I told her the story. She had a good chuckle as well.

Celeste asked me how long I thought she had in prognosis. We went through the blue book and checked off a few symptoms. According to the book, it looked like she had maybe four months or so. However, Celeste's abdominal girth had doubled in size in the past month, and she had zero bowel sounds on the entire right side of her colon and minimal on the left side.

I explained that she may have four to six weeks, but the will to live could extend the prognosis. Despite telling me that she was "ready to go," this would not be the case as I got to know Celeste over the next two months.

We agreed on a plan for three nursing visits a week; Monday, Wednesday, and Friday. Extensive pain issues and psychogenic pain would need strong case management from the beginning. Psychogenic pain involves psychological factors, anxiety, stress, and increased sensitivity to pain.[3]

---

[3] Dignity Health, "Psychogenic Pain is Real Pain: Causes and Treatment," https://www.dignityhealth.org/articles/psychogenic-pain-is-real-pain-causes-and-treatment.

She agreed to oxygen set up and Yonkers suction but no other equipment. There was no room to put the hospital bed in her bedroom as all the furniture and belongings were packed in tightly. We discussed placing it downstairs for when she couldn't go up and down steps. This was put on hold for a later time. She wanted more time to clean and reorganize things in the living room.

Her diet consisted of nutritious liquid soups and blended shakes. She was hyper-focused on the enemas for daily bowel movements. She said the gas pain and bloating were intense, and she felt she needed daily bowel movements for relief. Education was given on the number of calories she was taking in daily, which was from 500 to 800, and the number of bowel movements that should occur every week. We settled on a goal of three bowel movements per week. Celeste stated that, "I know if I stop eating, I will die much faster!"

Celeste's home had two stories filled with many possessions. She loved to shop and thrift. She was trying to organize things in totes and containers for Jacob, so he would know where everything was and what was in the boxes. I think Jacob was happy she was doing this so it would be easier for donations to be made after she passed.

Her bedroom was upstairs, and the bathroom was directly by the stairs. At first glance, this was a big concern for obvious safety reasons as she was getting weaker. If she took a tumble down the steps, it would end badly. Two days prior, she had a fall with no injuries. Having the baby gate at the top of the steps reassured everyone.

During every visit with Celeste, there was a notable beginning, middle, and end in how we carried out the tasks. I learned very quickly to surrender to her process, with boundaries, of course. When someone has OCD as a part of their mental practice, there is no turning the tide to suit your way.

Psychogenic pain is very real, and with Celeste, I believe it carried a high level of intensity along with her tumor burden. I started by incorporating the other modalities that I knew she would be receptive to since she embraced alternative therapy with herbals. She was quite amenable to massage therapy and prayer.

The visit began with vital signs and pain assessment. I documented the numbers and saved them on the computer. It was always important to do a count on the narcotics as her titration levels were weekly as the pain increased.

Celeste chose aromatherapy oil for back and neck massage. During this time, I gave her the opportunity to express her anxieties, things that weighed heavy on her heart, and unfinished projects. She was on a timeline to complete tasks, as she knew her days were numbered. As her emotions and tears increased, I offered to pray with her and for her. She was very strong in her faith and enjoyed this connection.

At times, Celeste would feel guilt or shame. "I just need to believe in His grace and what He did for me on the cross." Praying with her would relieve her anxiety for the time being. It's not all about the anti-anxiety medications.

After two weeks on service, Celeste started having a hard time swallowing. The medical director ordered liquid oxycodone for breakthrough pain. All equipment was now in the home, but she wanted nothing to do with the hospital bed. It remained downstairs. I think patients often feel that when they get into the hospital bed, they know their time is near. It is a big decision, one of surrendering to the process of dying.

She was ready to start the methadone, so the Fentanyl patches were removed three days later. She had gotten up to eight rounds of breakthrough of oxycodone per day, which was 240 mg daily. Her starting dose of methadone was 1 ml two times a day, 20 mg per day.

Celeste began using less fiber in her liquid drinks as it was getting harder to digest it. The routine of daily enemas continued whether successful or not. We were now up to 2 ml of methadone, six times a day titration over the course of 11 days. That is 120 mg per day. She also took Phenergan four to five times a day for nausea and averaged five doses per day of oxycodone (150 mg). The Ativan had changed to liquid concentration for easier preparation with pre-filled syringes and labeled in baggies. When she first started that at 1 ml (2 mg), it was too much, so she cut back to 0.25 ml at a time.

A few days later, she decided she didn't like how the Ativan made her feel, so she went back to melatonin for sleep at night. She had a loose stool with a magnesium drink since the enema didn't work, and her new goal was to "make it to Christmas!"

The next day was December 1st, and Celeste had a panic attack. The sisters were with her when it happened and called me right away. I instructed them how to put the oxygen on her and to give her a dose of liquid oxycodone to get her to calm down.

I made a visit, and we came up with a plan for moving forward. Celeste loved a plan! One of the sisters insisted that this be typed up and put on the refrigerator so everyone would know. The plan was as follows:

1. apply oxygen at three liters,
2. give a dose of oxycodone,
3. Call hospice nurse,
4. *Do not call 911,*
5. Pray with Celeste.

The next day was a routine visit, and I found Celeste in the hospital bed for the first time. She enjoyed being able to press the buttons for the head elevation and not having to use five pillows to prop up. She kept the oxygen on all the time now. Jacob had prepared several baggies with the dosage of 30 mg of oxycodone, which was 1.5 ml in a syringe. He labeled them to be given every four hours. This would help Celeste stay time-oriented.

The nausea was increasing, so Phenergan four times a day continued, and she started Prilosec. The methadone increased to 8 ml daily in divided doses, and oxycodone five times on average daily. It was time to start decorating for Christmas, which she did into the wee hours of the night.

Celeste did not want to stay in the hospital bed all day. She kept busy for short periods with activity. Afterwards, she would lie down to rest. She told me, "If I stay in the bed all the time, that means it's the end." A few days later, the methadone was titrated up to 10 ml per day.

Jacob and Celeste wanted to show me their shell collection from Hawaii. They enjoyed telling stories of their trips and showed me the wonderful craft projects they made from lovely shells from the shore. It was beautiful to see them review their life together.

Christmas was approaching fast, and the anxiety was escalating. We tried Lexapro, but that did nothing for her, so we stuck with the original narcotics of 12 ml per day on methadone by titration. I again discussed the Macey catheter as a better area for absorption of meds versus oral to the upper GI tract. Visible tumors were now appearing on Celeste's mandible and forehead.

I encouraged Celeste that it was her choice when she was ready to surrender to the process. Jacob had already given her permission to make the journey on several different occasions. She was determined to see Christmas as it was her favorite holiday. She forced herself to eat at least two bites per day with the liquid bone broth.

Two days later, her left foot and lower leg had four plus pitting edema. It was cool to touch, with no pulse palpable and red striation marks up and down the foot. We elevated it above the level of her heart, and Celeste was ready for the Macey catheter. There were zero bowel sounds present, and I asked her to please not put nutrition inside her as it would come back up.

The next day, Celeste decided to take the Macey catheter out herself and go back to oral meds. Christmas was eight days away. Her blood pressure was dropping, so she had to have standby assistance for any ambulation. The edema in the left foot went down to a two plus after some elevation, and the temperature warmed up again. The dexamethasone was discontinued, and she returned to low amounts of clear liquids.

As Christmas slowly approached, Celeste continued her interventions of enemas and sips of fluid to keep going. The sisters provided gentle massage to the left leg. The coccyx started to turn red. Celeste didn't like the Calazime cream because it turned her gown white. I asked Jacob to buy some boxer shorts to keep her gowns from discoloring.

On Christmas Eve, Celeste had a large bile yellow-colored emesis. I asked her to please stop drinking anything as her body was clearly rejecting it. She complied and asked for the Macey catheter again. The great thing about the Macey is that it is not sterile. So, for every practice run we tried up until now, I washed it afterward with soap and water and put it back in its container kit. I inserted the balloon with only 9 ml of water, not the full 15 ml.

Any more than that, and Celeste said it was painful in the rectum. She had no muscle or fat left on her thin body, maybe just a little on her thighs. All of the big interventions and hurdles we jumped over took time with Celeste. This is how she coped. She made the decisions for when she was ready.

I offered to put in a Foley Catheter on the day after Christmas, and she declined. She said, "I'm ready for the Lord to take me home." This time, her declaration was resolved, unlike the first time she spoke about this at the beginning of the journey.

Celeste had been on daily visits for a week. The weekend nurse attempted Foley catheter placement as it was getting too hard to roll and turn her. She was unable to get it in. It was too painful, and came out bloody-tipped, so a brief was applied. Her abdomen now had the appearance of being eight months pregnant with tumor burden.

In earlier conversations with Jacob, I told him what may transpire at the end with tumors of this type and how coffee ground-type emesis can come up. This is why I wanted a Yonkers suction present. I asked him to have dark towels ready the last few days by her bedside and to always keep her head elevated to at least a 60-degree angle. Jacob understood the instructions. But nothing can quite prepare you for when it happens, and it is dramatic.

Celeste's pain escalated, evidenced by grimaces and moans. She did not want to be turned. The medical director gave orders to apply two of the 75 mcg Fentanyl patches and methadone, 3 ml, five times a day (150 mg) via Macey catheter along with five doses of the liquid oxycodone, 150 mg. Celeste's eyes became glazed over, and her arms were reaching up toward Heaven.

The next day, her heart rate went up to 120 with 30-second periods of apnea, and oxygen levels remained at 97% on three liters. There was no urinary output for 48 hours. The following day, her oxygen levels dropped into the 80s. I visited around 11 am and encouraged Jacob to call if he needed anything. Celeste was comfortable at the time.

As I approached my next patient's home for a visit, Jacob called in a panic and said the coffee ground emesis had started. It was very disturbing to him. I reassured him what to do, and one of the sisters was present to help. I turned around and headed back to Celeste's home.

When I arrived, they had just finished cleaning her up and were applying a new gown. I went to Celeste's side, and she started to make noises like more was going to come up. We quickly got more dark towels in place. I honestly cannot say the amount that came out of her, but it was traumatic for even me to process. The Yonkers suction was no help because it was projectile and in copious amounts.

I prayed, crying out loud to God, asking to have mercy on this sweet soul and to take her home and end her suffering. And that He did. Celeste died with her eyes opening up on her last breath as she sat forward in my arms.

Celeste was on service for almost nine weeks. She made it to her favorite holiday of Christmas and shared it with the love of her life, Jacob. She was able to complete many projects that were so important to her. I titled this story "I Will Decide" for her because this was how we approached every intervention and every visit with all the details. I grew fond of her precision and the space that she needed. It's amazing what our patients can teach us if only we allow ourselves to soak it all in!

Hospice Highlights

- Complexity of this case: balance all of the symptoms, especially anxiety. Work within boundaries established mutually. Psychogenic pain is factual and critical to determine early in the patient's care.
- Treat all the categories of pain with the appropriate medication
- Importance of thinking ahead and preparing the caregiver and family for the active dying process, which may vary based on diagnosis. In this case, dark towels, washcloths, and Yonkers suction.

Source

3) Dignity Health. "Psychogenic Pain is Real Pain: Causes and Treatment." https://www.dignityhealth.org/articles/psychogenic-pain-is-real-pain-causes-and-treatment.

ONE IN A MILLION

I don't know where to begin with this unique story. There are so many things to say about this wonderful father and son relationship. Upon first meeting Conrad, he sat proudly in his hospital bed and was clearly the *king of his castle*.

He lived on the first level of his home, and his son Charles and his family lived upstairs. Conrad was 72 years old and had been on home health services before being transitioned to hospice. He was doing physical therapy for strengthening after a severe stroke. He was also having a difficult time with endurance and doing the exercises due to the residual effects of the cerebral vascular accident. This was intensified with the co-morbidity of advanced diabetic neuropathy.

Charles set an extremely high standard for caregiving of his beloved father that I had never witnessed before. He was meticulous, organized, and mindful of all the details as Conrad was completely bedbound. Devotion and patience were tactfully implemented in the day-to-day tasks. The bond between these two was truly authentic. Absolute love and humor were demonstrated.

I remember walking this journey with them in sheer amazement at the way they dialogued with each other and respected one another. You just do not see this kind of *unconditional love* every single day in a father-and-son relationship. A remarkable component in this story is that Charles was the principal caregiver for his father in his household.

I had to inquire further about their relationship and how it came to be. When Charles was 10 years old, his parents divorced.

Conrad had primary custody of Charles and his brother. He raised his sons with a strong German work ethic and may have been just a *little* on the authoritarian side of child-rearing. Charles would say, "I was a covert rebel and not an overt rebel." He learned how to walk the line. Above all, Conrad loved his boys through actions and deeds, not just words.

When Charles was in daycare and became sick with neurological symptoms of headache, fever, and pain in his neck, the doctors told Conrad it was nothing to worry about. Conrad saw that his son was not getting better but worse and advocated fiercely for further diagnostics and a spinal tap. It revealed meningitis, diagnosed just in time for treatment that saved Charles' life. This was one of many times in Charles's life that his father truly advocated for him and his brother. He genuinely loved his boys.

Unbeknownst to Charles, he was learning the role of caregiving growing up with Conrad as a single parent. Both boys had to do their share of the household chores. He learned early on that he had to be *responsible and to work for it.*

At age 14, he started as a dishwasher in a restaurant, then moved up into busboy and prep work. Later, he worked at a nursing home and underwent nurse's aide training. Adulthood brought commercial truck driving, and work as a safety officer in the oil fields. Every trade he learned *prepared* him for taking on the role of caregiver for his father.

Every member of our hospice team loved visiting Conrad. Our home health aide and I were scheduled for three weekly visits, and the Chaplain and volunteer participated regularly. It took a small village to ensure everything was attended to, especially when Charles had to go back to work after his six months of Family Medical Leave Act (FMLA) time was up. His work schedule would be two weeks at work and then two weeks at home.

Charles hired 24-hour-a-day agency help for the two weeks he worked away from home to ensure his dad was cared for properly. This was no small feat to accomplish. There were many issues with staffing consistent personal care attendants and managing their shifts, whether for 24 hours or multiple days at a time. Many items were put into place to make this happen: a video monitoring system, blood sugar monitoring, and daily phone calls to the agency to make sure they arrived and were performing tasks for Conrad's care.

Conrad had an extensive list of co-morbidities, including dysphagia, dysarthria, heart disease, hypertension, chronic pain, and diabetes mellitus. This played heavily along with his stroke symptoms. With the ensuing dysphasia and only taking in liquids, weight loss was occurring rapidly. This was shortly followed by skin breakdown on multiple areas of his body, which required a wound care regimen three times per week.

The most challenging part of Conrad's care was that it was 24/7. Charles stated that executing the routine every morning helped establish structure throughout the day. Creative checklists and staying organized were a necessity as the primary caregiver.

His pain was managed with a low-dose Fentanyl patch, liquid morphine for breakthrough pain, and Neurontin for neuropathy pain. We tried methadone since Conrad's pain was largely neuropathic in nature. However, this did not work well, as it had a sedating effect on Conrad. We continued with Fentanyl and morphine for pain management.

Over the eight months Conrad was on service, the pain meds were titrated about every two months and doubled in amount each time. This was needed for wound care pain, lower extremity edema, and general pain of being bedbound and over six feet tall. He required a Foley catheter and a Hoyer lift for bed care and bowel elimination protocol.

Conrad experienced several aspiration events with the dysphagia. The first few were mild, and he was able to clear the abnormal sounds from his lungs. But when the following event happened, I thought he was in the dying process as all of his vitals and respiratory system reflected it.

Charles was away for work. Conrad started to experience 45-second periods of apnea, and respirations were at six for three days in a row. His oxygen levels had dropped to 65% with oxygen on at three liters continuously. He slept most of the day, did not take in many fluids, and couldn't swallow his normal pills. His speech was slow, and he was withdrawing daily into deeper sleep. Edema was three plus in his lower extremities. After three days, I told Charles I didn't think he was going to pull through, so he came back from his work hitch early.

Well, I was wrong. Conrad slowly perked up when he saw his son and decided he wasn't quite ready to transition! Saturation levels rose from the 60s back to a healthy baseline of 97%, and he cleared the crackles and rhonchi sounds from his lungs. Conrad lived four more months after this event.

It never ceases to amaze me what people can withstand, and I really believe there is a choice when people are ready to leave their body. The process of surrendering from their physical existence is a timeline that one can truly participate in. Perhaps he wanted to make it to his 73rd birthday, which was one week after this respiratory event?

We fondly remember when his favorite CNA brought him an around-the-world feast of his beloved German foods to celebrate his birthday. He could only take a few tastes, but he embraced the presentation. Conrad pressed onward and made it to Christmas and into the New Year.

On a Friday, his oxygen levels were in the 90s, but he was maxing out on oxygen at eight liters, and his lungs were very coarse. I was on call Sunday when the call came in from the caregiver that Conrad's breathing was changing, and he was very wet sounding and congested with fluids that were starting to come out of his mouth. I arrived 15 minutes later. He was taking his last breaths.

We did our best to dry his mouth with cloths to have an absorbable mucosa for the morphine to engage properly. I applied morphine onto the green mouth sponges and inserted them into his cheek pouch to help the respirations be more at ease (his breakthrough morphine dose was high at 80 mg).

Since Charles was away at work, he watched his father's crossing over through the video monitoring system. He was able to say I love you one more time. I prayed with Conrad and asked the Lord to take him into his presence and bestow mercy as he transitioned. It was an honor to be with him for those last moments.

Afterward, I was a complete sobbing mess. I couldn't stop crying! The tears flowed for several hours. I had to call my favorite CNA to come and help with his personal care and to dress him. Yes, the bond is deep, tangible, and even more special the longer we get to know our patients and work with their families. It is good to cry, release the emotions, and to process as best we can.

Charles dealt with his anticipatory grief by mostly compartmentalizing it and detaching during the process of caregiving. However, he did have a few times of breaking down, crying, and engaging with his emotions. After it was over and he passed, Charles said it was a physical relief knowing he was not in pain anymore.

Years after Conrad passed, I asked Charles how he coped with being the primary caregiver. He said it was a substantial change transitioning from the home health side of receiving skilled help for his father for specific tasks to the hospice side, which was *all-encompassing*. He didn't feel he needed group therapy or special support after Conrad had passed because the hospice team had worked so dynamically well together for the eight months he was on service. The team provided support for both the patient and the son. There was a special working relationship between all the different disciplines of nurses, CNA, chaplain, social worker, and volunteer between Charles and his father. *It was unexpected, and he was grateful.*

Hospice Highlights

- Extensive organization & routine are required as a primary caregiver for someone who needs 24-hour care.
- Engage in the all-encompassing care.
- Detailed communication is necessary between all disciplines and the primary caregiver.

I'LL DO IT MY WAY

Driving cautiously down the windy road during a light snowfall, I took my eyes off the GPS as it no longer read my location, and the signal was gone. Time to look at the written directions to find my new patient. As foretold by the admitting nurse, "You'll probably go past the driveway because you won't see the mile marker due to the sharp turn in the road."

Of course, she was correct! I turned around and made a good running start to get up the unplowed, 70-degree incline driveway.

This was my first winter driving my new car, Silver Streak, an SUV with all-wheel drive and fancy buttons for extra traction. I thought I could downsize to this smaller-size car and be content with a lighter-weight vehicle. Sadly, I was mistaken with this assumption, as will be explained in *another* story. I prayed hard as Silver Streak begrudgingly inched her way up the driveway through ten inches of snow. I believe angels gently pushed from the unseen realm to get me to my destination.

I was greeted by a sweet silver-haired lady. Betty shouted at me from the top of the steps, "Come on up the stairs to meet George!" In the background, I heard George yelling, "Just come on up!"

George sat stoically in his favorite, very well-worn, brown recliner. His red robe over sweatpants would be his signature look for the months to follow. George was polite in his introduction, telling me he felt fine and wasn't having any pain to speak of. He explained the doctor found "potential cancer spots" on the lung, and he wasn't going to go through any treatments since he was too old! He was 88.

George had been diagnosed with prostate cancer with metastasis to the bone and had completed chemotherapy a year prior.

George's granddaughter, Cindy, lived on the first level of their home, and his son was nearby. They were busy with their work schedules, so my only communication with them was by phone for the first few months. I was concerned about whom would be caring for George when he started the active dying process, as Betty could not do so. Cindy said she would take time off work if needed. She worked as a personal care assistant.

I soon realized that Betty had dementia as she asked questions repeatedly and did not remember the answers. George kept a close eye on Betty, especially when she was in the kitchen cooking. During the first few months, George could care for himself, and go outside to smoke, but his energy levels were low, and he needed naps. He could run errands to get the mail and a few groceries. Initially, George only wanted once a week visits, but after a month in, I felt the need for more. I recommended that "With the swelling in your abdomen and feet, I need to keep a closer watch on these symptoms."

I offered to massage his legs, and he took me up on my offer. I've never had a patient refuse therapeutic touch. It is a wonderful way to begin a strong connection on so many levels. It helps establish trust as you spend time listening to your patient open up about their life. Allowing them to talk while you just simply hold presence and listen is irreplaceable.

As the weeks progressed, George's pain was minimal. He tried a dose of 0.25 ml of morphine. It really did nothing for his pain, which I expected as it was primarily neuropathy pain in his feet. He was not interested in starting a specific medication to target this pain. He declared, "That's too much fuss!" George was content with taking Tylenol to help the pain and didn't see the need for more drastic measures. At least he wasn't afraid to try one round of the liquid morphine, and I knew his response to it.

Initiating Lasix, a diuretic, helped reduce the edema in his lower legs. Part of his comorbidity list included heart failure and chronic kidney disease. During this time, George started to have dark-colored stools. He had a history of diverticulosis. He informed me that it would only happen once a day and that he wasn't too concerned.

I explained that the dark color indicated blood loss, and he wasn't bothered by this development.

As the months progressed, George told me his appetite was going away. Nothing tasted right or pleasing anymore. It didn't matter what he tried to eat, whether it was soup or something light, nothing was enjoyable. He did enjoy going out to smoke on his balcony. This was a ritual he didn't want to part with. So, I worked with George, not against him.

The doctor ordered Duo Nebulizers to help with his wheezing and rhonchi sounds in the lungs. This was likely due to the metastasis to the lung or the effects of long-term smoker's lungs. It didn't matter the cause; George wanted some relief with his breathing, so he would do the nebulizer treatment twice a day on average. He maxed out on diuretics for the lower leg edema and edema in his abdomen. After a few weeks, the medications weren't effective any longer.

After five months on service, it was early in May, and spring was in the air. The beauty of the birch trees were just beginning to display their new green tapestry for the season. George had called to cancel my Tuesday visit because the Episcopalian Chaplains were coming to visit and bring communion.

This was the first time they had visited since Covid began. I found this rather unusual as George never canceled any of my visits. I told him that was wonderful as he was getting ready for a big week of activity with his relatives coming up from the lower 48, arriving on Friday. They had plans to celebrate his birthday a month early. George told me he wasn't really looking forward to them making the effort to travel to see him. But he wasn't going to stop them from coming either.

On Wednesday, we were in the middle of our bi-monthly meeting of the interdisciplinary group when George called and said he was having a lot of pain everywhere and had taken one ml of morphine (20) mg and had no relief. I instructed him to take one more ml of morphine and headed to see him right away. I knew something drastic was occurring as George never had complaints of severe pain, and he had not taken any morphine in four months!

It was hard not to speed to get to George's home. I had no choice but to drive slowly due to the time of year we were in. A good portion of Alaska's springtime season is termed Breakup. This occurs when the final snow is melting, ice is thawing out, and the roads and driveways turn to deep muddy ruts! I put Silver Streak into Sport mode to get up George's driveway.

I found George sitting by the window in a different rocker chair, eagerly watching for my arrival. His face was very stoic, but he had a scared look in his eyes. I took his vitals and inquired where the pain was.

George was holding his abdomen and said it was all there, beyond a 10 out of 10 on the pain scale. I palpated the abdomen, and it was hard as a rock. I asked if he could walk to his bedroom, and we did so. It took about five minutes to get there, about 20 feet, as George held his belly for support and protection.

Once settled in the bed and after a few more back-to-back doses of morphine and Ativan, he still had no relief. I called our medical director, and he instructed me to insert a Foley catheter to rule out bladder distension and then to *shake the bed* while George lay flat. The catheter insertion was not possible due to extensive edema in the scrotal area. When I shook the bed, George hollered out in excruciating pain. Our medical director assessed that, most likely, peritonitis had set in. I told George he could revoke hospice and go to the hospital for assessment and diagnosing, but he adamantly said, "No."

I offered the hospital assessment because what was occurring was not anticipated in his normal declining process. What was happening was completely unexpected and very sudden. I explained we would need to medicate him well to get the pain under control with a Fentanyl patch and could use the Macey catheter for med administration. He agreed to this plan. I explained he would most likely go into a deep sleep and pass within a couple of days. George said he was ready to go and had lived a long life.

I explained to Betty what was happening. I think she understood at first, but then would ask again what was happening. I called the family to come home as soon as possible.

Meanwhile, our nurse practitioner, who was training in hospice, arrived to help. She wasn't able to insert the Foley catheter either. So, we applied a large brief and chux pad underneath. The Macey catheter was inserted without any problems. She brought the 100 mcg Fentanyl patch from the pharmacy and applied it to his upper thigh area. We stayed with George for a few hours until Cindy arrived. George was starting to drift off into a deep sleep at this point and appeared very comfortable.

The next day, when I walked in the door to greet Betty, she said, "I think he's still sleeping, but his hand has been up behind his head all night long, and it won't move." It was obvious George had passed sometime during the night as his right arm was in a fixed position propped up behind his head. His face was relaxed and motionless.

Even though George came on to service for metastatic prostate cancer, it was something else that ended his life. Peritonitis is inflammation of the peritoneum and is usually caused by a bacterial or fungal infection. Signs and symptoms include tenderness in the abdomen, pain that increases or gets more intense with sudden movements, abdominal distention, minimal urine output, diarrhea, and excessive thirst.[4] George had all these symptoms.

I believe George was ready to depart after receiving spiritual support from his church. The season of Covid took a lot of things from us. Still, when his chaplains were finally able to visit him in his own home and deliver the sacrament of Communion, he came to a place of peace and rest.

His body then surrendered to a process that had been building up quietly for some time. He also knew that his sweet wife of 55 years could not care for him, and he would have to rely on his granddaughter, which meant that she would quit her job for the time being. He chose to leave this earth before the family would arrive to see him one last time.

George did it his way!

---

[4] Johns Hopkins Medicine, "Peritonitis," https://www.hopkinsmedicine.org/health/conditions-and-diseases/peritonitis.

Hospice Highlights

- A hospice nurse needs a reliable vehicle that is compatible with their work environment.
- Early on, assess strengths and weaknesses of the caregivers in the household and those who come to help, like friends, relatives, etc. For example, if one spouse has dementia or is otherwise handicapped to administer the medications, other alternatives must be put in place.
- Tune in to what the patient says concerning potential treatments. It is their decision after the facts have been explained.
- Therapeutic touch with a patient can open doors of trust and communication.
- A patient's decline can occur more rapidly than anticipated, be prepared to take immediate action to inform family members of the plan of care.
- Often, a patient's choice is to avoid excessive personal contact with family and then departs suddenly. There are multiple reasons for this, but it's OK. They may prefer to be remembered in a more vital and vibrant way than their present physical condition.
- Understand the signs of Peritonitis: tenderness in the abdomen, pain that increases or gets more intense with sudden movement, abdominal distension, minimal urine output, diarrhea, and excessive thirst.

Source

4) Johns Hopkins Medicine. "Peritonitis." https://www.hopkinsmedicine.org/health/conditions-and-diseases/peritonitis.

SPRINGTIME

On a warm summer afternoon in late July, I arrived at the front entrance of Katy's home. As I opened the tall gate to enter the driveway, I was instructed that her mom's cottage was behind her home. I made my way along a winding path through a fairytale garden of flowers and beautiful rose bushes. I felt like I was in a trance as all my senses were transported to another time and place. I could have relaxed in this serenity for hours.

The end of the pathway led to a picturesque and whimsical cottage where Cadence awaited. The ability to grow beautiful gardens in Alaska is a testament to the character and personality of a soul with great patience and creativity. Cadence's passion for gardening was bestowed to her by her mother and passed on to Katy, her daughter. A generational love for cultivating timeless beauty was present all around me. Cadence loved to get on her scooter and go through the garden, watering the flowers during the summer.

Spring was a time of *great anticipation* for what was to come. I couldn't wait to meet the grand matriarch of the premises as I had heard so much about her!

Cadence was sitting in her recliner, ready for my visit. Oxygen was on, and her legs were propped up to help reduce the swelling. Cardiomyopathy was her primary diagnosis, with comorbidities of congestive heart failure and chronic obstructive pulmonary disease (COPD). She had a twinkle in her eye and a lively spirit that naturally invited one to get to know her.

I was helping the case manager with a routine visit and with inspecting a rash on her back for which she was taking Diflucan. The rash had a yeasty appearance, and the Diflucan seemed to be resolving it. Cadence had been on service for almost three months and on several rounds of antibiotics for urinary tract infections during that time. Before hospice admission, she had a hospitalization to correct abnormal potassium levels. After this event and a visit to the pulmonologist, the family believed it was time for comfort measures at home.

In December, I took over as her case manager with much delight. Cadence was 92 years old, had a cheerful personality, and was optimistic in her outlook to keep pressing onward. She enjoyed each day for what it would bring with family interaction, playing games, and often with her cup of coffee in hand. It was a challenge to get her to drink just water!

December's challenge brought an area of cellulitis on the elbow, which we treated with Epsom salt soaks, bacitracin, and a round of antibiotics per the family's request. It cleared up after ten days. Cadence was limited on which antibiotics could be used as she had multiple allergies. Often, meds that would work for most people would not work for Cadence. Katie had a condition called "Pseudocholinesterase Deficiency." This process affects how one breaks down muscle relaxant medications and can also cause an increase in sensitivity to other medications. I suspected Cadence, her mother, also had this with her long list of sensitivities and allergies to medications.

In January, she was on day three of an antibiotic for a urinary tract infection. She had a fall that night that resulted in considerable pain in her back and ribs, leaving a noticeable bruise. She slept heavily the day afterward. She only had one Tramadol for pain; however, her lung sounds were becoming more coarse with crackles, and she was declining rapidly with her oxygen saturation levels lowering also.

I updated all her children on her deteriorating status. I placed her on daily visits as she was on a trajectory of preparing to make her departure with the altered vital signs, the decline in mentation, and respiratory status. A Scopolamine patch was placed to help dry up the wet sounds in her lungs. This was her first time on this medication. Within 24 hours, she experienced hallucinations and anticholinergic syndrome.

SPRINGTIME

Even though it improved her lung sounds with saturation levels rising, the Scopolamine patch had to be removed. She had a few doses of Ativan to help with the anxiety and tremors. The on-call nurse came out one night as the restlessness was still present. She administered oral Ativan, which helped her relax and fall asleep.

It took five days for her to pull out of this event. Her PPS (Palliative Performance Scale) rose from 20% to 40%. Cadence's neurological status was back to her baseline. However, at times, she would experience underlying confusion. Her back and ribs were still tender to the touch, with some bruising and edema. She continued with as-needed Tramadol for pain.

At the beginning of this episode, we ordered the hospital bed and other needed equipment and placed it in Katie's home. We were expecting Cadence to move up there quickly as she was declining. However, Cadence had other plans. She wasn't quite ready to depart this earth! We left the equipment in place for when the transition would happen.

Katie reminisced that after this fall, the pace increased in her overall decline in status. Cadence moved into Katie's home three weeks later. She needed more help with all her ADLs (Activities of Daily Living). Living in Katie's home also provided much easier and more frequent sessions with her son-in-law, Tom, who played her favorite games and allowed her to keep her Yahtzee winning streak going.

Another UTI was brewing as symptoms started to escalate. Managing Cadence's UTIs involved antibiotics due to the severity of her symptoms, with nausea, vomiting, and hallucinations. It would bring relief for a short time, then the cycle would repeat. However, in this episode, she was experiencing nausea, vomiting, and pain in her gallbladder area.

It was difficult for her to keep the antibiotic in her system. She had a history of gallbladder disease with calculi. We suspected this was flaring up again with the symptoms that presented.

She tried reducing fat in her diet to help with flank pain to no avail. She continued taking prednisone for the ensuing rashes that presented on her body, with oral Benadryl and low-dose Xanax for the anxiety at night. Edema in the lower legs increased, and some weeping of fluid started in her toes. Her beloved CNA provided a lymphatic massage to help with the discomfort, which Cadence thoroughly enjoyed.

At times, Katie would get frustrated and wished she had not corrected her when her Mom's behavior was off, and she was confused. Trying to be sensitive during the altered thought process moments was challenging. She loved her mom dearly and wanted to hold on to more time with her and do what was possible to keep going forward.

In a casual conversation, Cadence told Katie that she would not be here during springtime to help with the flowers and planting. Katie didn't realize she was trying to prepare her for what was to come.

One day in April, Katie called and said Cadence was more confused. She didn't want to wear her oxygen, her lifeline. It was off when I arrived, and her saturation levels were in the 80s. We reapplied it, and back up to 90% it went. Her shortness of breath was managed by oxygen.

The family wasn't quite ready for morphine to come into the care plan. The possible reaction of this medication was unknown. The flank pain was increasing, so she took more tramadol and Xanax. The next night proved to be more eventful. Cadence hallucinated as she got up from her bed and walked through the house. She had incontinent episodes and then cut up her oxygen tubing. Cadence had done this a couple of months before when she lived in her cottage. At that time, Katie removed all the knives and scissors from the kitchen.

She told Katie she didn't know why she was still here and was ready to go to be with the Lord. Katie felt that in her mom's mind, the oxygen was preventing her from leaving this world. She had been oxygen-dependent for four years.

A couple of days prior, her son-in-law, Tom, had tested positive for Covid symptoms. Katie then followed. We swabbed Cadence and her test results came back negative. However, it was apparent she was symptomatic. We consulted with the medical director as to whether it was best for Cadence to stay home if Katie and Tom couldn't take care of her since they were sick. Everyone agreed a hospital stay was not desired as no one would be allowed to see her due to the strict visitation policies. Cadence did not want to die alone in a hospital.

Then a miracle happened, and a dear friend of the family came to town. The timing of her visit was not planned but sent from above.

SPRINGTIME

She had wonderful caregiving abilities, and since she had recently had Covid, she was fine with this responsibility. Her hired caregiver and friend, Jess, also increased her hours to help. Jess had become like family over the months with her overnight and alternating day shifts to help care for Cadence.

During the week that followed, the caregivers tended to Cadence as her oxygen levels dropped, and she continued to decline. Later, I asked Katie how she embraced the grieving process. She told me everything was beautiful and peaceful. "Jesus was here."

Two days before she passed, Cadence had great moments of clarity with a surge of energy. The family sang hymns, with some family members on the phone and a few in person. The on-call nurse visited to place the Foley catheter as she couldn't void anymore. The nurse explained very precisely what was happening with her organs shutting down step by step. Their anxiety was relieved with the delivery of this information.

On her final day, the Macey catheter was placed for ease of morphine administration to help Cadence's breathing be calm, and a low-dose Fentanyl patch was placed. Cadence's heart rate slowly decreased in beats per minute as she drifted into a deep sleep.

As her heart beat its final moment, I believe her first embrace was with her Creator, whom she loved with all her heart. Her *anticipation* was encountered with a beauty incomparable to our earthly knowledge as she leaped into His *springtime* garden.

Hospice Highlights

- Infections can cause the end of life in non-cancer diagnoses such as UTIs, cellulitis, and viral upper respiratory infections.
- Work with your families to achieve comfort care in the home setting. Be flexible with the medications.
- Acknowledge when people who are oxygen-dependent are ready to remove their lifeline.

SOARING WITH EAGLES

My eyes filled with delight upon my first meeting with Violet. She lay in her hospital bed, her delicate 90-pound body taking ownership of her new home. Her silver-colored hair was propped up in a high ponytail as she talked with spunk in her step. Her deep hazel eyes and vitality lit the room with an effervescence that continued with every visit for the next eight months she was on service.

Violet was admitted to hospice after the doctors told her they could not do surgery on her broken hip since her lung disease, Chronic Obstructive Pulmonary Disease (COPD), was in the final advanced stage. The surgeon told her she most likely would not wake up from the anesthesia. She agreed to care and comfort measures and to move into her daughter Rae's home.

In her mind, this was a temporary plan. Violet's goal was to get strong, walk again, and move back into her *own* house. After all, at 88 years of age, she had been living independently for the past 37 years since her husband's passing.

I'll start off by saying that the majority of people who have broken a major bone, whether it be a femur, hip, or humerus bone, will die within five to ten days if there is no surgical intervention. *Of course, Violet was an exception to this rule and too many more rules that would follow in the months ahead.*

I was quite shocked the day after admission when I observed she was able to turn side to side and log roll without significant pain. Her oxygen saturation levels were 88 on oxygen at five liters continuously, and noticeable mottling discoloration was present on both knees. I wasn't sure if Violet was going to pull through.

To help provide relief of extra exacerbation with turning, we decided to place a Foley catheter. Attempted would be the better word. Insertion was successful; however, no urine came out until an hour later. Then she started to bypass urine onto the pad in small amounts as well as flow into the catheter bag. I explained to Rae that sometimes this can happen, and we needed to monitor the amount.

By 10 pm, it was leaking heavily. Violet said, "I can tell I'm peeing!" I removed the catheter, and we decided to continue to use small, tabbed briefs. In my opinion, Foley catheters are either a blessing or a curse. I usually like to give it a week or so to see what issues may arise and if they are conquerable. In this case, it was a hard NO.

Premedication with small amounts of morphine a few times per day was important to relieve the discomfort of being bed-bound and the isolated pain of the fractured hip, especially before giving bed baths. Violet was quite confident she could manage to be in briefs with this condition. We developed her plan of care moving forward. Violet's mantra was: "I'm going to get stronger and get up and walk again!"

The relationship that Rae and Violet had was quite special. It was an honor to be a part of their journey and see the dynamics that unfolded in the months that followed. At times, I felt like I was watching two best friends banter back and forth, and at other moments, watching the daughter/mother duo wrestle with daily routine intricacies.

I set my schedule for three times a week to help support Rae as she was the primary caregiver for her mom. It usually boiled down to one child that takes on the burden of being the sole caregiver. Our Certified Nurse Assistant (CNA) played a vital part in helping Rae and Violet manage her personal care. Everyone who met Violet fell in love with her on day one.

It was one week after hospice admission when her skin became affected with a pressure injury starting on the coccyx. Over the next few months, the stage one pressure injury advanced to stage three. It would temporarily close over and then open up again. By her first recertification period at three months, we tried to dangle and sit up on the side of the bed to get stronger, but dizzy spells took over with weakness. They were short-lived exercise events. Violet was determined and kept the ongoing dialogue, "I'm going to get up and walk again!"

I really did feel obligated to try and help her work through the experience of sitting on the side of the bed for strengthening, especially after she told me the story of when she was 14 years old and went through an appendectomy with no anesthesia. She lived in Italy, and this was during World War II. She told me there was no anesthesia. They just had to remove the appendix. She stated, "I lived through it!" When I heard this story, I knew we were in for a fun and wild ride.

Our CNA managed to get Violet up to the shower a couple of times while on service. She was refreshed after the event but then exhausted the next day. Bed baths became the norm for her routine after that.

Six months in, she experienced an upper respiratory infection with mild fever. Rae wanted to do a round of antibiotics. She stated, "I want my mom to live as long as possible."

Our nurse practitioner confirmed that since it was not brown or dark sputum, most likely, it was just a viral infection. The plan was to increase nebulizer treatments and take Tessalon Pearles Rx, which resolved the infection. A second pressure injury had appeared on the mid-spine.

Rae needed a break as the primary caregiver, and our plan was to have Violet go to our contracted facility for a respite stay. Nevertheless, the pandemic was going through another surge, and Rae requested to keep her home and have daily nurse visits while she went out of town. Another family member stepped up to help out and stay with Violet.

As the autumn season approached, Violet faced another challenge. She needed to spend time with her son, who was diagnosed with a terminal illness and was advancing into the final stages. The family came together and shared some precious moments. They captured the moment with photos of mother and son lying side by side, one in the hospital bed and one in a recliner chair.

A few weeks later, the pressure injury on her tailbone, which had been toned down in color and closed over, suddenly turned dark purple/black. A Kennedy's ulcer had presented. This was a hard conversation to have with Rae. I explained that her mom was on the final path to her journey home. Sometimes, it's hard for families to absorb this concrete information when they've been walking the road month after month, doing everything to give the best care possible to their loved ones. And then this happens.

Kennedy's terminal ulcer is a specific type of pressure ulcer (also referred to as pressure sore, pressure ulcer, or decubitus ulcer) that is characterized by rapid onset and rapid tissue breakdown. The Kennedy ulcer was named after Karen Lou Kennedy-Evans, the nurse who discovered the medical condition. Like most pressure injuries, Kennedy ulcers are believed to develop due to poor blood circulation that results from unrelieved pressure.

However, Kennedy ulcers differ from other pressure injuries because of:

- Rapid onset, a wound may go from a blister to stage 4 within hours
- The wounds tend to grow downward, as opposed to horizontally
- The wounds are most often located on the sacrum
- Wounds are almost exclusive to the elderly population
- The wounds are usually irregularly shaped, frequently described as pear-shaped
- Death occurs quickly, as many patients succumb to Kennedy ulcers within 24-48 hours of their onset[5]

The treatment options for people with Kennedy ulcers are limited due to rapid development and progression. Consequently, most treatments for Kennedy ulcers are focused on providing pain relief. It's important as a hospice nurse to become familiar with this early in your career so you can educate families on what this means. It is part of the preparation and teaching of end-of-life care.

---

[5] Nursing Home Law Center, "What is a Kennedy Terminal Ulcer," https://www.nursinghomelawcenter.org/what-is-a-kennedy-terminal-ulcer.

From my experience, when Kennedy presents, end of life occurs within five days. Rae received the information well and called the family together to spend time with Violet. The priest was called in for prayers, and in good Italian fashion, much food, laughter, and tears were shared over the following days.

When I visited that Friday, it was day three after the Kennedy's ulcer appeared. The house was full of many family members as they were celebrating Violet and had prepared her favorite Italian dishes. She could only handle a small taste, but the aroma of fine food permeated her bedroom. The priest would come at night for final blessings and prayers.

I was off for the weekend and knew I had to say goodbye to my Sweet Italiano. I hugged her tight, and with many tears, I told her I loved her. She responded, "I will love you forever!" She had a peaceful look of gratitude as she knew where she was going with all the confidence in the world.

I drove away, trying to process my emotions. I stopped to see my sweet barista daughter as she made me a coffee drink. She knew I was having a rough day when I pulled up in tears. I only hope that one day, if I ever need help from my baby girl, it will be like the relationship Rae had with her amazing Mama!

Sometimes, we don't get to process for very long before we are off to our next patient. We must strive onward, "Plod On," as my dad would say. As I drove to my next visit, the Autumn leaves were dancing in the wind, some trying so hard to stay attached to their branches, their place of belonging.

This somnolent summer had been excessive with the amount of rain we received. We felt robbed of this short season and were now heading into a long winter too quickly. The beautiful country road curved around the hay fields, and a gorgeous Bald Eagle appeared out of nowhere as the grey clouds parted and patches of blue revealed themselves.

It flew above my car, maybe 50 feet away. I could not keep pace with this majestic eagle. It followed me for several hundred feet. The Heavens quickened my heart that this eagle was like Violet. She had run her race strong with exuberance and vitality. *We just couldn't keep up with her anymore.* It was her time *to soar*, and soon, she would be in His presence. Violet ascended into Heaven two days later. She was prepared and ready to take flight.

Hospice Highlights

- Develop your patient's plan of care; tune in to their goals.
- Identify when antibiotics can be beneficial or not and teach caregivers the purpose of antibiotic therapy.
- Distinguish when Kennedy's ulcers appear and clarify to families what this means in the active dying process.
- Make time in your day to process your emotions, compose yourself, and press onward.

Source

5) Nursing Home Law Center. "What is a Kennedy Terminal Ulcer." https://www.nursinghomelawcenter.org/what-is-a-kennedy-terminal-ulcer.

THE PAUSE

It has been one year since I began the adventure of creating this book. During the first five months, the inspiration was intense, and the thoughts and stories flowed easily. The motivation I felt while writing *A Tale of Three Men*, my first story, was remarkable. Then came a time of drought.

I just couldn't get back into the writing process and focus. I struggled to research the chronology of events from the chart and blend information about how the stories played out. My thought process was very fragmented. This was a dry season with no inspiration. I didn't know why, so I put it aside for a while.

I recall crying out to God, 'What is wrong? Why have the words stopped flowing when I know I need to write this book?' I felt the words in my spirit, 'You are in a pause, and a pause is coming.'

I didn't comprehend what that meant until March 1st. I was transitioning my empty nest by helping my daughter move into her first apartment. On the last trip down the steps with absolutely nothing in my hands, I slipped and fell on the snowy, icy final stair and probably skipped a step.

I don't know how it happened. However, I do vividly remember hearing three loud noises, *snap*, *crackle*, and *pop*. The next thing I knew, I was curled up on my left side on the snowy ground. I lifted my right leg and saw my ankle dangling in the opposite direction. I had horizontal striped compression socks up to the knee, so the visual was quite disturbing!

My daughter, Bella, came quickly to hold me and put a blanket around me. I told her to call 911 immediately! My son, Simon, wanted to get me out of the cold and inside. I yelled, "No one is touching me but the EMT guys!"

The first phone call I made was to my boss. I told her what happened and wanted to be sure someone would take care of my patients. I didn't know how much pain medication I would receive, and I didn't want to forget to let work know I wouldn't be coming in tomorrow. I was in shock.

The first call my daughter made was to my sister, Beth, who lives in South Carolina. She had just returned home from Peru, leading a medical mission with her nonprofit group, Esta Lucecita. Beth was known for her quick action and strategic planning, and before long, the inner circle of the family knew of my mishap. I intentionally did not call my mom that night as I didn't want her to worry. But she managed to hear about it very early in the morning. By then, everyone was praying for me.

It took ten minutes for the ambulance to arrive. They asked how to get me up, and I responded, "I don't know, you guys are the experts, you decide!" They attempted to snuggly hold my leg against the stretcher, which did nothing to help the pain. Going over the snowy bumps on a cold stretcher to the ambulance (about 15 feet) was the most intensely wicked pain I have ever experienced. It was worse than transition in childbirth or passing kidney stones.

I begged and pleaded for them to move slower. They bargained with me to move even quicker, and the reward would be IV Fentanyl in the ambulance. I quickly agreed to that intervention! Once in the ambulance, they gave me 175 mcg of Fentanyl through a swiftly inserted IV. The relief was immediate, and I started to relax, and the pain started to lessen. The ride to the hospital took another ten minutes.

Upon arrival, the ER doctor looked at my oddly shaped foot, whipped out his phone, and said, "I have to take a picture for future reference. We haven't seen a break this bad in a long time!" Well, leave it to me for my first broken bone to be not just one, but three, a Tri-Malleolar fracture: tibia, fibula, and malleolus. The ER doctor called it a dirty break.

That visual was not very pleasant as my mind tried to figure out what that meant through the haze of Fentanyl fog. I remember the med tech said, "We need to cut off your tennis shoe. Is that ok?" I agreed, and they cut my shoe off and my pant leg up to the knee. So much for my new tennis shoes, which were designed to help with my plantar fasciitis!

The view of my ankle rotated to the right at almost a 90-degree angle was a ghastly sight to everyone, myself included. But I was receiving excellent pain meds and didn't mind. I was also still in shock.

After x-rays, the doctor saw increased swelling, and the bone was almost ready to project through my skin by the medial malleolus. The foot and ankle were pale purple-blue and cold to the touch. He commanded his staff to move quickly for the reduction before the bone would pierce through. Then they gave me Ketamine.

Talk about an amazing experience. It was a unique out-of-body feeling, as if I was looking down from above and watching the staff and doctor reduce the bones. It felt like a minor cracking of knuckles.

At this moment, Simon walked into the room. Bella said he looked pale as a ghost when he saw the reduction take place. He declared many times later, "I could never be a nurse or work in the medical field." It must have been traumatic to see his Mama experience such harsh physical trauma and realize her mortality was not forever.

I went home that night, enlisting my little bird, Bella, to come back with me to the home nest. I couldn't let her fly just quite yet. She asked, "Why would the universe let this happen?" Many answers were yet to be discovered on this journey. Moderated rest began, and five days later, the first visit to the orthopedic doctor occurred.

My sister flew up right away to supervise the first part of my recovery and initiated the plan for caregivers to follow. X-rays showed the bones were starting to separate, the reduction was not holding, and a fracture blister had developed on the medial malleolus. It was interesting to watch the staff grab other staff members to see what was on my ankle.

The doctor called in the casting personnel, and they gently wrapped my leg for transport to another room for wound care. This involved popping the blister, letting it drain, and then cleaning and applying Silvadene and securing it with a partial cast splint to tide me over until the next day. I was not familiar with a fracture blister. One of my nursing cohorts with ortho experience told me that fracture blisters happen in only 3% of all cases. That explained everyone's fascination with the blister that looked like a purple egg!

The doctor said I needed surgery as soon as possible and that he would add me to the schedule at the end of the next day. He needed to place an external fixator to keep the bones in place while the swelling reduced and the fracture blister healed before surgery for internal hardware. As Bella helped me to bed that night, tears finally flowed for the first time. This was all so overwhelming. The orthopedic surgeon's words that I would not be able to go back to work for 14 weeks were beginning to sink in.

As a single woman, this was hard to comprehend. The severity of my accident was beginning to be absorbed in my mind and heart. It's remarkable how your body protects you initially from the impact of trauma until you are ready emotionally and mentally to begin processing. I had been functioning in the mode of shock and denial with the magnitude of the situation.

After 18 hours of taking nothing per mouth, the external fixator was placed. My sister poignantly asked the surgeon if I could have a nerve block before the external fixation, and the doctor said he would assess the pain after the surgery. I didn't get the nerve block, and his reasoning didn't make sense to either of us. Needless to say, the pain was beyond severe.

I stayed overnight on the med surge floor so I could receive adequate pain control with IV meds. I needed IV Dilaudid every two hours throughout the night. I switched to oxycodone tablets before leaving the hospital to return home. A few days into this experience, I knew I would need a hospital bed and walker. It was too difficult to get in and out of my bed or to prop the pillows to create the elevation needed for above the level of the heart. I left the hospital with crutches initially, and before long, I had a walker, stroller, wheelchair, bedside table, and bedside commode. Having the ease of pressing a button to get into the proper position for leg elevation was wonderful, and altering positions in my upper body alleviated kidney aches and pain.

It's hard to describe the feeling of the air mattress. It felt like a creepy crawly sensation at times when the bubbles alternated the air pressure. I wasn't a big fan of the feeling. I knew it was needed to help my skin condition, so I kept it on the bed. But I now understood why some of my patients didn't like the air mattresses, especially if they were light sleepers.

I was thankful my equipment company from work set up the hospital bed and air mattress by my big window looking out to the meadow. This would be my view for the next 16 days while I recovered.

My sister's friend in Michigan, who worked for an ankle and orthopedic specialty group, strongly reinforced that bedrest was absolutely critical at this juncture and compliance was an integral part of the healing process. *It was not a suggestion; it was mandatory.* I appreciated her advice, as the orthopedic group I was seeing didn't drill that home to me as strongly as she did. Thankfully, Alaska displayed some beautiful sunny days during this time. The vitamin D coming through my sliding glass doors and picturesque sunsets at night helped keep my spirits positive during the days of pain. My view was inspiring as the meadow was lined with snow-covered trees trying to shed their winter coats. March and April presented what we call Spring 1, Spring 2, and Spring 3; maybe it's really here now, or maybe not.

It is hard to describe the type of pain experienced during external fixation, but I will try. Multiple stainless-steel pins were drilled into several bones to keep the bones externally in place until the internal hardware surgery. It was a combination of neuropathic pain and somatic pain in nature. It was a feeling of fire, burning, and stabbing pain with deep internal pressure. At times, it was intermittent. At other times, it was rhythmic in nature, and a buildup would occur to a crescendo of needing narcotics, Tylenol, Advil, and a muscle relaxer.

The pain during the "cleaning" of the stainless-steel pins was horrific. Those nights after the cleanings, the pain was the worst. One night, I awoke to my leg having spasms. It looked more like a seizure, and I had to hold my leg down to get it under control. Managing the pain was a struggle.

The experience of the external fixator and being on bed rest was the most painful part of the journey. For the first two weeks, I was taking pain meds, two oxycodone 5 mg tabs every four hours, a muscle relaxer at night (sometimes during the day), and Benadryl and melatonin to help me sleep.

I recall one night, a friend visited for almost three hours. We got caught up in laughter and amusement as she tried to teach me to crochet. We all passed the blanket around and took turns working on it. Amidst storytelling and fun, my mind was completely distracted from the pain. As soon as she left to go home, the pain immediately soared up to a 6/10 scale. There is something to be said about distraction therapy!

Along with the narcotics came constipation, of course. I took multiple stool softeners, including Senna-S, Calm drink with magnesium, Bisacodyl tablets, and suppositories, and ate prunes and fresh fruit. I drank two liters of water every day, plus a triple-loaded collagen drink with one liter of water to increase wound healing. I was getting in plenty of fluids. This regimen was simply not enough.

My daughter, who thankfully is medically inclined with a caregiver's heart, had to give me enemas. This was one of many personal care tasks I would need help within the upcoming weeks. Narcotics and immobility contributed to slow motility. The dependency of needing help for everything while on bedrest with bathroom privileges was all-encompassing. Enduring so many things being stripped away from you all at once is overwhelming. I couldn't work, couldn't drive, couldn't prepare a meal, couldn't walk without devices, couldn't bathe myself, and couldn't take care of my pets. I couldn't live on my own for the first two months. The intense pain with the external fixator and dependency on so many people to keep me alive and functioning brought me to a place of complete brokenness.

There was ample time for quietness and reflection. This could produce good fruit or not. *I had a choice to make in this process.* Could I walk through this with grace and the needed fruit of patience? Could I find the blessings in all of this, or would I choose to be bitter and angry that it even happened?

So many friends, family, new church friends, co-workers, and hospice family/friends visited me during this time. The meals provided and house chores that needed tending to were indeed a special gift. The compassion and generosity with sacrificial monetary giving and making time in their busy schedules to spend time with me was truly humbling. It truly was above and beyond my expectations.

One of the nurses I worked with started a GoFundMe to help with medical expenses, etc. I was reluctant at first, but then I agreed. I was so blessed by the many donors. Something amazing I witnessed was that those who had the least to give financially were the ones who received tenfold more in monetary blessings when they gave an offering to help me. The return to them happened within a few days of their giving. It was beautiful to see when hearts give sacrificially, the blessing of how God returns, which is rather exquisite.

I experienced God's extravagant love and would never be the same! Love truly is patient, kind, and not self-seeking. The actions and deeds demonstrated by those who cared about me confirmed the real fruit of faithfulness, as well as the many prayers from those near and very far away.

A big sacrifice was made by both of my nieces, Maddison and Carly, who flew up from out of state. They each spent a week caregiving for their Aunty with much kindness. Bella juggled her college and work schedules to help as much as she could. Simon helped with the outdoor chores, shoveling, and chauffeuring.

In this place of brokenness, I learned to live through what I knew would be temporary. Were any of these things I experienced similar to what my patients went through? I felt like I understood maybe a glimpse of what they go through now. I hoped I would become a better nurse as a result of my experience.

Sixteen extremely long days later, I was ready for surgery number two. I almost had a setback two nights before surgery. I came down with the stomach flu. Thankfully, it was mild. Bella helped me with ambulation as I felt dizzy and did not need another fall with the Ex-Fix on. Nothing was going to delay this surgery. I was so done with the Ex-Fix and the intense pain and taking narcotics around the clock. The fracture blister closed over nine days after it was presented. I believe the triple load of Xyngular collagen powder played a key role. That, along with lots of prayers coming my way as well.

The medical staff at the orthopedics office commented that the healing taking place was impressive and faster than they expected. I was ready for the internal hardware surgery (Open Reduction and Internal Fixation).

This time, the anesthesiologist was right there to give me two nerve blocks, one under the knee and one in the ankle area. The surgeon told me that I would experience arthritis in this ankle in the future, and the hardware would most likely be permanent. The surgery took longer than planned due to the metal plates not fitting and having to be shaped to size to fit properly.

After the surgery, the surgeon then told me I would most likely want to get the hardware removed within six months due to the tight fit of all the plates and pins/screws that were placed. They would cause discomfort and pain; how much would be the question? I went home to recover.

The morning after surgery, I awoke to the hospital calling to follow up. When I looked down at the ace wrap over the leg, there was blood coming through on the medial ankle. She advised me to call the ortho doctor, and they had me come in to see what was going on. Normally, my follow-up would have been 12 days out. After inspection, it was concluded the stitches were intact, and this was a small bleeding response. A new half cast/splint was applied.

Coming out of the nerve block took around 70 hours. It was a 24-hour block, so that was interesting. The sensation and pain were unique as that wore off, feeling pins and needles and heaviness. At least I didn't have to take oral pain meds every four hours during those first days after surgery.

Three days later, during a visit to check incision sites, everything looked very good. Every visit to ortho included another X-ray of the leg bones to monitor the progress. Thirteen days after the surgery, the surgeon was very pleased with the healing. He asked, "Can I trust you?" I answered, "Of course, I'm a nurse, and I can obey orders." He said we could skip the cast and go right to the boot. The only time it was to come off was for a shower. I readily agreed. I was absolutely shocked that I was able to skip a step on the leg apparel.

The referral for physical therapy was sent, and I began that 18 days after surgery, ten days ahead of the original plan. Since I couldn't bear weight yet, I thought PT would involve the rest of my muscle groups as I was severely deconditioned from 5 1/2 weeks of bed rest. That was not so!

Lymphatic massage and gentle range of motion exercises and stretches were on the agenda for the right ankle through the edema and gridlock of the ankle bones. Two times a day, I repeated the exercises, and on every visit, I would get a new set of movements as they kept building upon each other. Those initial stretches performed by the PT were off the charts with deep pressure pain.

Coming off narcotics was not as hard as I anticipated. The intensity of the pain was lessening but changing in character. Nonsteroidal anti-inflammatories and Acetaminophen were a part of my daily regimen for the months to follow.

A dear friend told me, "Sometimes God has to allow a hard stop to happen in order for His work to be done." At this point in the journey, I had experienced brokenness literally on so many levels. The portal was opened, and the words started flowing once again. The focus, clarity, and recall of the details of the hospice stories I needed to write presented beautifully. Composing the stories and usually going to four appointments per week between PT, chiropractor/massage, and orthopedics actually kept me busy. Spending time with old friends and cultivating new friendships was an enormous added blessing.

Every day had a purpose.

I found time to simply rest and had time to dream. I dreamed of what my future might look like now that I had launched my young adults. The last time I had this much time off work was maternity leave, and that certainly was not rest. But rather a time of surrendering to the concept that your life is not your own anymore by bringing new life into the world and experiencing the love of parenting.

For eight weeks, my lower leg and ankle had felt like they were not a part of my body but rather a foreign object. There are no other words to explain it. Then the big day had arrived, as Bella told me that morning, "May the Fourth be with you!" It was May 4th, the day for my first steps and learning how to walk again. Walking on water, that is, and yes, I asked Jesus for help! Well, taking my first steps in the 90-degree therapy pool water.

Being in the therapy pool was wonderful. Of course, you feel only 30% of your body weight from the exercises. I was able to follow through with the different movements. Then, it was time to come on land and try to walk.

At first, my PT said, "Try with one crutch on your left, move it forward, then step in with your right leg." Well, that was about impossible as my hip caved inward. I tried with two crutches, which was much better for support. I was sent home with four exercises to do twice a day. The boot was to be on for the next two weeks as I gradually transitioned to tennis shoes.

That afternoon, we packed Bella up, and she flew back to her apartment. I made sure I could take a few steps with the crutches and not fall, so I felt okay to be alone. Then, a harsh reality set in the next morning when I tried to do the exercises. This was ten times harder than the luxury of the therapy pool! I started with floor mat stretches in every direction to prepare my body for daily weight-bearing exercises.

The next day, discouragement flooded me; apparently, I needed a good cry fest. I've learned over the years that it's not good to ignore the need to cry; you should just surrender to the process and embrace it. I could only do two of the four exercises according to the instructions. My right knee would give out from weakness and pain.

I took to Amazon and found a good stationary bike with support for the back that was reasonably priced. It arrived at the end of the week. I knew going to PT two times a week would not be enough, and I needed more strengthening equipment in my home that would be easy on my right knee. The knee was a big area of pain and tenderness during the initial weeks of walking. I felt like the clock was ticking as it was less than six weeks to be functional to go back to case managing in the field. I requested my supervisor to not have any on-call as I would need a few months to rebuild stamina. It would be challenging enough to handle the 40-hour work week.

After four days of weight bearing, I had follow-up x-rays at the orthopedics office. The physician's assistant (PA) said to take the boot off and only wear tennis shoes. I was surprised again! So much for the full two weeks in the boot.

She was very emphatic, "We have to get you walking!" After I left the office, she called me to declare, "I forgot to tell you, the sooner you can ditch the crutches and go to a cane, the better off you will be." That was overwhelming to hear as I could not tolerate weight yet on the right side.

After a full seven days of partial weight bearing on the right side, I had a turnaround. I believe it had something to do with soaking in a very hot tub with three cups of Epsom salts. The next morning, the swelling had gone down, and I was able to take about 30 steps with one crutch. I was shocked. Even though the swelling had mostly resolved prior to weight bearing, it all returned with a vengeance now that I was training all the muscles, tendons, joints, and bones again to walk. The nightly Epsom salt hot baths became a ritual.

I met with my nurse practitioner six weeks into this process, and I requested a Dexa scan to see if this injury might be osteoporosis-related. She did not bring it up during the visit; I had to advocate for myself! This was my first fracture, and this was a severe one. My surgeon said this was the second worst break one could experience.

It took multiple calls to get this order because she didn't process it initially. It never ceases to amaze me in our medical world how much you must be your advocate, constantly pushing for what you think would be beneficial. After completing the Dexa scan, I received part of the results. I had osteoporosis. The med tech would not tell me the percentage number score. That would be discussed during my next appointment, two weeks out. However, the NP wanted to call in a prescription for Fosamax!

Well, that about did me in. This was no way to inform your patient of a new disease. Either give me all the information on the phone or call me in for an appointment, preferably less than two weeks out. I changed to a new practice with a functional medicine approach.

I searched for meaning in all of this. If I had not had this severe fracture occur, I never would have found out I had osteoporosis at the age of 51. This type of fracture, Tri-Malleolar, is not a typical osteoporosis fracture. Those usually occur in the hip or wrist. It was good that I now knew this information to treat this disorder properly. Typically, insurance will not pay for the diagnostics until age 65.

With progress comes regression. I had overdone it on my treadmill at home, and the next day, I started to feel some sharp pain in the tendon. I had a pool session that morning and tolerated it fairly well. The next day, I could not follow through with the pronation motion of a full step. I was back to using two full crutches and could hardly place my right foot down. I took it easy all weekend and only did stretches that didn't involve the left half of my foot. I focused on using my little weights for upper body and thigh exercises and core work. Three times a day, I doused my foot with coconut oil, frankincense, and peppermint oils. I massaged my foot, stretching in multiple directions, and used the massage gun on the lowest setting for the calf muscle, followed by propping up on the pillow. It was three steps forward and two steps back.

It was an intense six weeks of PT and exercises at home. My physical therapist said that people with this type of break usually walk with a limp for several months after PT is completed. I appeared to be healing better than most of his clients. One PT out of the whole group was very accurate and honest in her assessment that the full recovery process would be one year once ambulation started and the metal was removed.

Before I knew it, it was time to go back to work on the first day I was allowed to drive. I had to use a cane for my first 12 days, and I walked one step at a time, very methodically, into patient's homes when stairs were involved. Thankfully, I had new nurses to train those first few weeks. We worked together on the patient's physical care, as I could not do it by myself at this point. During charting back at the office, I would elevate and ice the ankle, which would get me through until I returned home and elevated and iced again.

My summer was filled with work, taking walks, and doing exercises to build strength. I managed a few short hikes in the mountains on easy trails. There's nothing quite like being in the Hatcher Pass mountains surrounded by green alpine tundra, crisp air, wildflowers, and blue skies to replenish the soul. Rebuilding stamina and endurance would take many months, and the one-year prediction from the PT would prove to be accurate.

I decided to get the metal removed at the 7-month mark, as I was experiencing achiness in the tibia bone that was noticeable with every step and tightness in the ankle. It felt like a rubber band was growing tight around the ankle daily. We experienced an extremely rainy and cool summer. The surgeon said the colder temperatures worsen the achiness. Winter was fast approaching, and it was time for the final surgery!

One screw had to remain in place as the CT scan revealed the bone was healed, but there was a depression in the malleolus. My Surgeon consulted with an ankle specialist who confirmed one screw should remain. The rest of the metal was removed, except a tiny portion of a small screw from the plate had adhered to the bone. This recovery was a breeze compared to the other two surgeries. The nerve block was sufficient for pain control, and I needed only a few pain pills the next day.

Once the stitches came out, I used the cane for a few hours. Building up strength again was the goal. I was thankful I did not have to depend on the cane. I started with short walks on the treadmill, slowly increasing my time every day. The achiness was gone. However, some tightness remained in the joint. Time would tell the full healing process. Eight months after the hardware removal, I estimate ankle mobility to be at 90%. It was worth getting the majority of the hardware removed!

During the mobility recovery, I worked closely with my new provider, doing blood tests to check calcium and magnesium levels, 24-hour urine, and many other lab values every two months. This included diagnostic tests that insurance would not cover: Metabolomix and Dutch testing. I was diagnosed with idiopathic hypercalciuria, magnesium deficiency, estradiol deficiency, oxidative stress, and multiple nutrient deficiencies.

My gut was not absorbing the nutrients I was taking in, so I started on digestive enzymes and several supplements. I was shocked because I didn't have typical symptoms of digestion issues. The most difficult thing I had to give up was coffee. Caffeine hinders the absorption of calcium. Drinking decaf was not advised due to how it is processed with chemicals. I didn't realize how addicted I was to coffee; the smell of coffee, the process of making espresso in my beloved espresso machine, and the effects of energy at my fingertips. I had been consuming close to 450 mg of caffeine daily.

I tried to do HRT, hormone replacement therapy, for several months. The side effects were too much, including weight gain and severe abdominal distention. I embraced all the other modalities to reverse the osteoporosis diagnosis. After six months, my NP ordered the NTx blood test. This test measured the breakdown of fragments of collagen byproducts released into the bloodstream when bone tissue is being broken down. The levels came back within the normal range and the bone loss had stopped. The functional medicine approach was working, and I would not have to go on prescription medication as the side effects could be quite severe. This regimen would be a lifelong discipline!

The Pause is credited for the near completion of this book. It took one more year for a few final stories and several edits. I understand now that beautiful things can come to fruition from a state of brokenness. Surrendering to the process and giving it the ability to flourish was the foundation.

THE CEILING IS THE LIMIT

It was a beautiful, sunshine-filled day as I drove to my new patient's home through the mountainous, curvy roads. I waited until the afternoon to see her, so the roads were plowed from the previous day's snowfall. The drive through the Chugach Mountain pass had many twists and turns lined by scant guardrails requiring full attention. One wrong move, and I would be taking flight to the next realm! Pumping the brakes often to keep speed under control, I would quickly take in a few glances to my right side to absorb the beauty of the jagged peaks submerged in white.

I was looking forward to meeting Lily, as she was a retired diploma nurse. I knew she would be teaching *me* new things. I believe the best nurse my generation has ever learned from was the Diploma Nurse. Their education was a solid three years in the hospital setting. The clinical hours they earned outnumber today's BSN by a huge margin.

When I entered the cabin, her husband, Jack, first offered me a cup of hot tea. I graciously accepted this on a cold winter's day. Lily was in her tiny room, propped up in the hospital bed with beautiful, long, silvery wavy hair decorating her pillows. Her left leg was wrapped in a sheet for support like a sling. I had never seen anything like this before!

We shared a cup of tea, getting to know each other while being warmed by the crackling wood stove. Lily had been diagnosed with kidney cancer ten years prior. It was an encapsulated tumor and stage one. She chose to do active monitoring with no treatment. She said the pros outweighed the cons. She did not want to do chemotherapy and put that "poison" into her body. She knew she could have several years before it spread, as kidney cancers often do not advance quickly when diagnosed early at stage one.

Lily wanted to have quality time as she had just retired from nursing at age 55. Her passion and hobby was gardening. She loved to spend countless hours outside during the long Alaskan summer days. She tended to her greenhouse and flowers all around her cabin, nestled deep in the woods alongside Jack.

Three months prior to coming on to service, a CT scan verified she had a pathological fracture in the L1 disc of her spine and a right rib fracture. Lily knew it was now time to ask for more help with hospice care as she had recently suffered a fall, which resulted in the fracture of her left femur. She was now bedbound, and all care was performed in the bed. Jack needed help as turning Lily with her left leg wrapped and slip sheet was becoming very hard on his back. She had developed a crafty way to maneuver her left leg because she didn't like the brace they provided her with when the fracture occurred. She had Jack wrap the entire left leg cradled in a sheet and wrapped in a sling style. We used the slip sheet maneuver to turn her from side to side with bed care.

Lily embraced the entire team and welcomed the aide, our CNA, who bathed and provided foot care. She enjoyed visits from the chaplain for spiritual support.

Upon admission, our medical director reviewed her current pain management routine. She rated her pain 3/10 initially with a combination of neuropathic and deep somatic pain. Lily described the pain as deep, sharp, stabbing, burning, gnawing, and aching. Her lower back and left leg were the primary sources. Lily had been on MS Contin three times daily for time-released control and taking oxycodone 15 mg for breakthrough pain on an average of three times a day. Lily agreed to try a different narcotic to specifically treat the neuropathic pain. It is critical to be thorough regarding pain assessment. The way the patient describes the pain helps steer the hospice team in the right direction.

Since Lily's pain was neuropathic and somatic in nature, she started on methadone 10 mg/ml concentration, 1 ml two times a day. Methadone usually takes 72 hours to take effect, so she stayed on the MS Contin until three days into the conversion. It took one week for the relief to occur, and then Lily rated the pain as 1/10. Lily had also been on a low dose of steroid to help with the bone pain, Dexamethasone 2 mg once a day. She was not on a proton pump inhibitor, so the medical director started her on Omeprazole to help with any stomach discomfort while on the steroid.

Over the next 2 ½ weeks, we worked on the bowel regimen by adding Lactulose and Senna S. This turned out to be a good combination. Pleased with the results, Lily's appetite picked up again. She was eating three small meals a day and enjoying treats her neighbors brought.

Lily was adamant that she did not want a Foley catheter. I asked at least once a week, but she always declined. She was now having an increase in pain, taking oxycodone for breakthrough pain six times a day. Lily knew it was time to titrate up the long-acting medication, methadone. But she didn't give the green light until two days later. Methadone was scheduled at 1 ml three times a day.

It is important to give your patient choices in all of the elements of care. They are losing independence every day on so many levels. Empowering them with decision-making is critical.

Four days later, Lily's left foot was turning blue, and mottling started. The edema was still 4 plus since admission on the entire leg. The dorsal pulse was very weak, and the temperature of the foot was very cool to the touch. We were concerned a blood clot may be forming.

I gave Lily the choice, "Do you want to try and treat this with aspirin therapy and see if it helps or just monitor?" She said she was not ready to die yet, so the medical director ordered Aspirin 325 mg two times a day.

Then she started to experience pain in the pelvic region, so methadone was titrated up to 2 ml three times a day. I encouraged Lily to try liquid morphine instead of oxycodone for quicker relief during breakthrough episodes. She was ready to do this, and it was an easy transition.

At this point, I asked if I could visit three times a week instead of two. She readily agreed. She also asked if I could type up a spreadsheet for Jack to write in and keep track of medications. It was getting harder for her to document in her journal, and she needed to turn this responsibility over to Jack. It was hard for a nurse to relinquish control of the documentation, but Jack would do anything for his beautiful bride.

Two days later the left foot improved as the blood clot symptoms diminished. It wasn't blue anymore, and the temperature was normal, so she continued with the aspirin therapy. She was, however, feeling a little loopy with the methadone titration. This sensation went away after a few more days.

A few weeks prior, I measured her leg for a different type of leg brace to support the pathological fracture. What arrived was a bit cumbersome. Jack showed me all the tools he had in his shed, which was quite a collection. He said he could modify the brace to fit Lily better.

He also showed me the stash of supplies of canned goods from their garden and food items. He enjoyed showing me Lily's final work, which she had produced in her garden the past summer. They were well prepared as they lived many miles from town. Alaska only has a one-week supply of food and staples in the grocery stores. Due to our isolation, it is quite common for folks to have a few months' supply of dried or canned goods in their pantry, as well as a freezer with moose and salmon.

Lily faithfully wore the leg brace for three hours a day to keep her leg aligned. Five days later, the pain increased again to a 4/10. Methadone was titrated to two ml four times a day. At times, Lily would have nausea and take Zyprexa to help alleviate this symptom. She taught me about how they would administer meds back in the "olden days" when it came to nausea. She said, "Rectally is not the only route, you can give meds vaginally as well." That was the first time in my career I had ever heard that!

Lily took 1 to 2 mg of Ativan at night to help her sleep as the pain levels were increasing. Later that week, her lungs presented with wheezing sounds. She was saturating in the high 90th percentile and had oxygen available to use when she wanted it. I believed lung metastasis was presenting.

That weekend, Jack called the on-call nurse because Lily was having urinary retention and bladder spasms. Still, nothing happened when Jack put her on the bedpan, and there was nothing in the brief. She was ready for the Foley catheter, and it brought her relief. The catheter would stay in for the duration.

On Monday's visit, Lily's pain was climbing again. She rated it 7/10. A few weeks prior, I asked our medical director if I could get a Rx for a Fentanyl patch and have this ready since Lily's pain was by far one of the most intense scenarios I had seen in many years. She also lived 45 minutes away from the pharmacy, and that was on a good day if the roads were plowed. I wanted to be proactive with her pain management.

A 100 mcg Fentanyl patch was placed transdermally. Jack administered all the meds as Lily's sleep had increased greatly, and she was drinking only small amounts of fluids; food intake had stopped altogether. She was not having difficulty swallowing, but as death approached, the body did not need food as it was too cumbersome to digest and evacuate when all systems were slowing down. Around four hours later, the Fentanyl kicked in, and her pain level was down. Jack said she was able to sleep with Ativan.

The next morning, Jack called while we were in an interdisciplinary group meeting. He said Lily was screaming in pain, and he had given several rounds of meds, but nothing was working. I could hear her loud cry in the background.

It took me 40 minutes to get to Lily's cabin in the woods. It was impossible to drive fast through the mountainous, curvy road. I had only seen a pain crisis like this once before in my career.

When I arrived, Lily was hollering in pain and completely inconsolable. She said it was her right kidney. It felt like stabbing and burning. The pain would come in rhythmic waves. She looked like a mother in transition before the baby would enter the world. I called our medical director, and he told me to give her meds every five minutes until she was comfortable and to apply a total of 300 mcg of Fentanyl patches. I gave 1 ml of Ativan, 2 ml of morphine, and 2 ml of methadone by mouth every five minutes. Lily was still able to swallow.

After 30 minutes of no relief, I asked the medical director if she could go to the hospital for a GIP (General Inpatient) admission. GIP is one of the four levels of care that hospice can provide. This level of care is specifically for when symptoms are not manageable in the home setting.

He informed me the hospital was full, the ER was full, and if we did send her there, she would be waiting in a hallway for a room. Lily did not want to go and die in the hospital. She made that extremely clear. I kept giving the meds, and we prayed that God would help ease her pain. Lily was wearing oxygen at three liters per nasal cannula. Her oxygen levels were 99% at the beginning of this pain crisis. It took one hour and 45 minutes for Lily to go into a quiet rest. At the end of this pain crisis, her oxygen levels were still 99%. If we took the oxygen off, she would drop to 85%.

In summary, that was a total of 840 mg of morphine, 420 mg of methadone, and 42 mg of Ativan given by mouth to get Lily's pain crisis under control. There is great truth in the concept of pain medications to treat the pain related to the dying process. *That the ceiling is the limit.* Everyone's body is different in how they process pain medications. One must also take into consideration that when cancer is eroding the organs of filtration, whether it be the kidneys or liver, higher doses of medications may need to be administered. Lily's story was not complete yet.

The next day, Jack settled into the routine of giving 2 ml of morphine and 2 ml of methadone every six hours by mouth. Her pain was at a 1/10. Lily's son was present and helping with her care. He had not been around in the weeks prior. Three days later, we were at the 9-day mark of no food intake and morphine for breakthrough every two hours. Her oxygen levels were at 93% on three liters, with fine crackles noted in the lung bases. But Lily still had unfinished business. She had not told her nursing friends that she had terminal cancer.

Jack called them to come by so Lily could say her goodbyes. This was the closure she needed, and she put it off until she was ready. They were not able to come until two days later.

At this point, the pain was escalating. Methadone was up to three ml four times a day. Saturation levels dropped to 88%. It was too difficult to turn and reposition her in the bed. Bloody urine was coming through the Foley catheter. We kept irrigating it daily to keep it flowing.

The next day, her saturation levels rose to 99% on three liters of oxygen. Lily was having 25-second periods of apnea. I still don't understand how saturation levels can rise when respirations are lessening. She was not going to leave this earth without a little bit of feistiness.

The following day, the Foley catheter was completely clogged, and flushing did nothing to open it up. It was changed out, and minimal bloody urine resulted. The next day, Lily's heart rate went up to 140 and her saturation levels were at 96%, still on oxygen. Her temperature was at 103.9, and she could not swallow anymore.

A Macey catheter was inserted to give her Tylenol to keep her temperature down and avoid possible seizure activity. The Macey made it easier for all medications to be given. The methadone remained at 3 ml four times a day, and morphine 2 ml every two hours. She was in a complete coma.

The next morning, Jack called me to come as her breathing patterns were changing quickly. When I arrived, I held Lily, prayed with her, and asked God to take her home as she had run her race well. She was ready for complete healing. Lily died in my arms a few minutes later. Her husband of many decades was by her side and faithful in all aspects of her care until the very end. I was honored this tender-hearted diploma nurse waited for her nurse to arrive and be with her when her spirit left her body.

Lily died eight days after that incredibly intense pain crisis. She was on hospice care for a total of two months. I learned so much from this beautiful woman. She had the will to live until everything was completed. She made her body hold on for a few more days until she could say goodbye to her nursing friends.

During those last weeks, her son, who had not been a part of her care, came back to her and helped as he could. This meant the world to her. She felt her son's love for the final time. What a beautiful gift he gave to her.

Hospice Highlights

- Understand the different types of narcotics and adjuvant medications that go for each category of pain so you can communicate clearly with your medical director or attending MD.
- In the home setting, oral meds or meds given via Macey catheter may have to be given in very short increments to resolve the pain crisis. This is very different than if IV meds were available. The hospice nurse must be comfortable following through with these orders from the medical director.
- Remember the rule of titration. When taking two to three doses per day of breakthrough medications, long-acting medication needs to be initiated. Also, increase the long-acting med when consistent breakthrough meds are taken, usually three times a day on average. (MS Contin, Fentanyl patch, methadone)
- Integrate emotional and spiritual support with pain management.
- Anticipate needs ahead of time if the home is not close to immediate response for escalation in pain symptoms. Have prescriptions on hand if appropriate.

ADDENDUM

Become proficient in the knowledge of different types of pain with hospice patients. These include:

- Nociceptive pain, which includes Somatic (bones, muscles, connective tissue)
- Visceral pain (internal organs)
- Neuropathic pain (nervous system)
- Psychogenic pain (psychological factors include the exacerbation of pain)
- Anxiety, stress, and increased sensitivity to pain

Learn to recognize the signs and symptoms of pain:

- Verbal expression (moaning, groaning, crying)
- Facial expressions (grimace, frowning, clenching teeth, rapid blinking, tightly closed eyes)
- Behavioral changes (agitation, restlessness, withdrawal, depression, confusion, easily angered)
- Physiological changes (increased heart rate, increased systolic blood pressure, perspiration)
- Physical actions (rocking, fidgeting, pacing, resisting care, guarding body part when turning, rigid posture)

- Focus on quality, quantity, and severity, and learn the trigger words. [6,7]

TRIGGER WORDS

- Somatic: pain with movement-bones (cramping, aching, sharp, and gnawing)
- Visceral: internal organs (deep squeeze, ache, pressure)
- Neuropathic: nervous system (numbness, tingling, electric, stabbing, burning)
- Psychogenic: complex with psychological factors (stress, anxiety, depression)[8]

CLASSIFICATIONS OF MEDICATIONS

- Anticonvulsants (Tegretol, Dilantin, Depakene) (Neuropathic pain)
- Try-Cyclic Antidepressants (Amitriptyline, Nortriptyline) (Neuropathic pain)
- Corticosteroids (Dexamethasone, Hydrocortisone, Prednisolone) (Adjuvant for Somatic & Visceral pain)
- NSAIDs (Diclofenac, Ibuprofen, Naproxen) (Adjuvant for Somatic & Visceral Pain)[9]

---

[6] Continuagroup. "Hospice Pain Management." *Continuagroup.* https://continuagroup.com/article/hospice-pain-management/

[7] Samartin NJ. "Hospice Pain Management." *Samaritan NJ.* https://samaritannj.org/hospice-blog-and-events/hospice-palliative-care-blog/hospice-pain-management/

[8] Continuagroup. "Hospice Pain Management." *Continuagroup.* https://continuagroup.com/article/hospice-pain-management/

[9] Hospice Management." American Family Physician. https://www.aafp.org/pubs/afp/issues/2014/0701/p26.html

- Opioids include the following:
  - Tramadol (mild pain) (1/10th as potent as morphine)
  - Hydrocodone includes Acetaminophen (moderate pain) equal in strength to morphine
  - Morphine and oxycodone (moderate pain) (oxycodone is 50% stronger than morphine)
  - Hydromorphone (moderate to severe pain) (5-10x stronger than morphine)
  - Fentanyl (moderate to severe pain), long-acting 80-100x stronger than morphine
  - Methadone (severe pain) Neuropathic and Somatic pain (3x stronger then morphine)[10]

Source

6) Continuagroup. "Hospice Pain Management." *Continuagroup*. https://continuagroup.com/article/hospice-pain-management/

7) Samartin NJ. "Hospice Pain Management." *Samaritan NJ*. https://samaritannj.org/hospice-blog-and-events/hospice-palliative-care-blog/hospice-pain-management/

8) Continuagroup. "Hospice Pain Management." *Continuagroup*. https://continuagroup.com/article/hospice-pain-management/

9) "Hospice Management." *American Family Physician*. https://www.aafp.org/pubs/afp/issues/2014/0701/p26.html

10) Drug Rehab. "Opioid Strength." *Drug Rehab*. https://www.drugrehab.com/addiction/opioid-strength.

---

[10] Drug Rehab. "Opioid Strength." *Drug Rehab*. https://www.drugrehab.com/addiction/opioid-strength.

TILL DEATH US DO PART

We were in the middle of an unusual Alaskan heat wave, temps in the high 80s, and very low humidity. The normal temperatures during summertime average in the 60's. As I knocked on the door, I was greeted by Harold, Janet's husband. She was the patient I was meeting for the first time. Harold was 91 years old, and Janet was 96.

I couldn't believe my eyes as I saw Janet sitting at the kitchen table, methodically eating lunch. Meanwhile, Harold was in complete respiratory distress, trying to catch his breath with audible wheezing while arching his shoulders. He was dressed in a long-sleeved flannel shirt, which I'm sure didn't help the situation.

He stood five feet away from me while he propped himself up and clung to the wall. My first thought upon seeing Harold was that I was going to have to call 911 or do CPR if this respiratory effort persisted. This was not the way you wanted your first visit to play out, having to code the spouse!

There is a reason I am not an ER nurse; I do not thrive on these types of adrenaline-fused scenarios. And to boot, I was training a new nurse on the hospice side. Thankfully, she was a pro and not alarmed by what she was witnessing. I barked out orders as she worked alongside me to get Harold comfortable as quickly as possible.

I asked him to please sit down before he collapsed so I could get an oxygen reading. He was saturating at 87% on room air and very pale and grey in color. I asked him if he wanted comfort measures like his wife and to be kept comfortable at home and not have to go to the hospital for treatment. He readily agreed, saying, "I don't want to go to that damn hospital ever again!"

I called his doctor, who fortunately was one of our medical directors, and he ordered admission to hospice. He knew Harold was appropriate for hospice care since he had end-stage COPD diagnosis. His previous doctor's visit included discussing oxygen in the home, but Harold was not ready.

I called the admitting team to load his stats into the computer, and then Harold signed the paperwork as I ordered oxygen for delivery as soon as possible. The durable medical equipment company provided a full setup and a nebulizer machine in one hour. He had an antiquated nebulizer, so he received a new one with a different medication (Duo-Nebulizer), which is more effective at opening the airway than plain albuterol. With the oxygen on at two liters and a nebulizer given, Harold started to breathe a little easier, and oxygen saturation levels began to rise to the mid-90s.

Janet's daughter, Laura, provided primary caregiving. Laura didn't feel Harold needed morphine right away. Oftentimes, people have preconceived ideas and knowledge about morphine and what it means at the end of life. I worked with her and Harold because he wasn't ready either to start taking a narcotic. I don't believe Harold had ever taken medication like this. He was a strong-willed, stubborn, hard-working Alaskan man. I wasn't going to push.

I educated them with frequent, gentle reminders that there were comfort meds in the home for when he would desperately want relief that oxygen alone could not deliver. The choice was his. We are creatures designed with free will.

Ten days after admission, Laura told me she thought Harold was ready for morphine as the duo nebulizers and rescue albuterol nebs weren't working. Harold agreed. We started at 0.1 ml (20 mg/ml concentration) morphine dosage (2 mg), a baby dose. It didn't provide enough relief, so 0.2 ml was given, which was a better dose. Adding lorazepam liquid at 2 mg/ml concentration for anxiety was beneficial as well, but we kept the dose at the very small level of 0.1 ml, or else he would get loopy in his thought process.

His respiratory effort was not as labored, and he was able to talk without getting winded. At this point, Harold was continuously wearing the oxygen at three liters. If he took off the oxygen, he would desaturate into the 70s. He was also placed on low-dose prednisone at 5 mg daily, but after ten days, no benefit was seen in his symptoms. It was evident that morphine played a much more significant role in helping with the severe air hunger he experienced. So, the prednisone was discontinued. With encouragement, Harold would pre-medicate for the air hunger before any exertion was made, and then he could tolerate it better. He was not 100%, but it was better than medicating afterward.

At age 17, Harold and his brother traveled the long road to Alaska in 1947. This was the first year the entire Alaska-Canada Highway was opened to unrestricted travel. He met Janet on a double date at a golf course, and they married and had two daughters.

When asked why she only had two children, Janet told Laura, "That's just what you did then!" Laura has fond memories of her mom's free and tough spirit as a strong Alaskan woman who took care of the home front while Harold was away working for the summer. Harold did carpentry work and guided hunting trips. The kids would often tag along and stay in a camper or cabins while visiting their dad on job sites.

Laura had vivid memories of her mom snow machining as she enjoyed "catching air" during the adventures. She said, "Mom had a happy-go-lucky spirit with no fear and was very hard working. She truly enjoyed her gardening and flowers." I think her phlegmatic personality attributed to her long life of 96 years. Harold specifically told me he chose to marry an older woman because women live longer than men, and she would be there to *help* him.

According to Laura, Harold had a more controlling personality and was inclined to be in charge of Janet. She tended to serve him in their approach to married life. As Janet had declined over the past several months, Harold was losing control on several platforms. He was losing his wife, as she just didn't care anymore with dementia advancing, and his own health was declining. He was losing the ability to do things independently, with his lung capacity deteriorating.

Back to my first patient, the other spouse! Janet was admitted to hospice for end-stage dementia. Over the previous six months, her decline had been advancing. She experienced a fall that resulted in a pubic ramus fracture and resulted in a three-week hospital stay. No surgery was needed. When she came home, she received physical therapy, occupational therapy, and continued wound care for her heel.

She used her walker somewhat, but then another fall occurred. Eventually, she became wheelchair-bound. She was not responding to the PT and OT, and no further hospitalizations were desired, so Janet transitioned from home health to hospice.

Laura lived a block away and wanted to give her parents as much independence as possible. She set a daily routine of when to come over and get her mother dressed and in her wheelchair for breakfast and then transfer to her recliner chair. She would go back and forth during the daytime to provide care for her mother. Harold would call in between if anything was needed or for any problems.

After one month on service, Janet was carrying along steadily. She needed wound care to the heel three times a week for a pressure injury and continued to eat. She could feed herself, but she needed total assistance with all her other activities of daily living.

One morning, I received a panicked call from Laura right before 8 am. Harold was on the commode and couldn't get up. He felt like he had fire stuck inside of him. Oh yes, I forgot to mention what had transpired with that little symptom called constipation. I will make a long story short. Harold suffered from constipation but was only willing to take one senna every other day.

I knew it wasn't enough stool softener because of the amount he was eating and not being physically active like he used to be. I could see his abdomen slowly getting larger in circumference. I explained we would have to do an enema if the senna wasn't working. He delayed it until the next day, which resulted in the crisis call.

Why was it that Harold attracted dramatic entrances to his house? As I barreled down his driveway and up the steep hill, a mama moose greeted me and her twin calves. They stood there right by his porch, acting like they were guardians of the property. I couldn't call Laura for help to shoo them away because she was standing by her dad at the commode!

I waited a few minutes, and they didn't budge. I got out of my car slowly and went to the trunk to get my supplies, not making any sudden moves in their direction. I didn't want to get caught in between them. Finally, they disbanded their security efforts, and I quickly ran up the steps into the house.

I had given Harold choices and he made them. Now, I had the privilege to make the choice, which was called the enema! Digital removal was first because he was completely blocked in the lower rectal vault. Harold's air hunger was also so severe he had dropped to the mid-70s. Getting him off the commode to his normal bed for the removal and enema was extremely difficult. After the procedure was done with a few rounds of morphine, he was more comfortable and calmer.

I had a straightforward conversation with Harold as we had established this connection the moment I met him in respiratory distress on day one! Harold was starting to transition. I explained to him he was on a trajectory to go to the next realm within weeks, probably less, as his lungs were telling us they were completely done. Harold acted surprised and said, "Really, that soon?" I said, "Yes, Harold, your lungs are entirely worn out, and they can't keep up with the rest of your body and mind even though you are very strong-willed and determined."

I explained it was time to get into the hospital bed for safety so we could do all the care in the bed. He agreed and didn't argue with me anymore. I thought he would be obstinate, but what he had gone through that morning scared him. Harold feebly walked to the hospital bed, winded, as I supported him with his last earthly steps. I got him settled in with side rails up for safety. I wonder what emotions his heart was feeling with that last walk.

Laura called her sister Ann, who lived on the West Coast, with an update on Harold's status. Ann had been up to visit a few weeks prior, but Laura felt she needed to give her the opportunity to come again if she wanted to help. Ann arrived four days after Harold was bedbound.

The day after becoming bedbound, Harold's palliative performance scale was 20%, with minimal bites of food and sips of water, and he was sleeping most of the time. Laura was concerned about Harold being "sedated," which would lead him to not being able to eat despite her feeling that he might be hungry. He would awaken but fall asleep before he finished a few bites of food.

Education was given on end-of-life signs and symptoms. We discussed the balance between keeping Harold comfortable with medication and keeping him awake and alert enough to eat and the purpose of food during the dying process.

One of Harold's friends came to visit the next day, and he told his friend, "I am going to fight this…dying." Harold kept his word. He didn't suffer from severe terminal agitation; he just had a hard time surrendering to the process. Usually, COPD patients will go fairly quickly when they start transitioning, but not Harold!

Laura and her sister reassured their dad several times that it was okay to go and reassured him that Janet would be taken care of.

I inserted a Foley catheter on the first day Harold was bedbound. Still, after four days, he was having several problems with spasms and leaking. Then, I couldn't even irrigate it because it was blocked, so we went with briefs and insert pads for incontinence. The next day, Harold moved into a semi-responsive state. When he rolled and turned in bed, his sats dropped to the 80s at five liters of oxygen. Morphine was given at 0.25 ml 6 plus times a day, and low dose fentanyl at 12 mcg helped with discomfort and shortness of breath.

He only drank fluids on the fourth day, and on day six, a small purple Kennedy ulcer was starting on the coccyx, so it was padded up with a foam dressing. He reached the mark of nine days with no food before he passed. He experienced his surge of energy that day as he requested several different drinks and drank them all. He spent the night mumbling and talking to people in the room all night long. His chatter kept both daughters awake as he wouldn't stop talking. Laura recognized his brother's name, and when she asked Harold about him, he nodded yes, saying that he was in the room. All his siblings had passed many years prior.

On the day he transcended, his breathing pattern changed several hours prior to fast, shallow breathing. Laura gave him 0.25 ml of morphine every hour to help his respirations to settle down. She was reluctant to give more. The mottling started in the knees; however, his O2 sats stayed in the low 90s, which was amazing.

Laura left to take a break at her house while Ann was on duty. She was on the porch looking in when she noticed he wasn't breathing anymore. Harold died in the presence of his bride of 66 years in the hospital bed next to him. This is the way Harold wanted it to be.

Laura was close to her dad and lived next to them for many decades. I believe he felt it would be too emotionally hard on her if she was present in the room at the very end. There truly is a choice when people are ready to leave their bodies. This is the last physical earthly decision Harold made.

I explained to Laura and Ann that his oxygen saturation levels would likely gradually drop. Of course, Harold had to prove me wrong, and that did not happen! Harold made the earthly departure his way, in his timing, with both daughters not present.

There was no time for Laura to process her sadness of losing her father as her caregiver duties continued with Janet. Her grieving process was postponed for some time to come. The feeling of numbness and thoughts of "Did I do anything to hasten his passing?" crossed her mind for weeks following.

Two days prior to Harold becoming bedbound, Janet had a neurological event, and it appeared to have been a Trans Ischemic Attack (TIA) mini-stroke. Or she may have suffered from heat exhaustion as we still were in the middle of the "heat wave" in the high 80s of dry heat and low humidity. With most homes not having air conditioners, simple fans had to make do. Laura also covered the large living room windows with dark blankets to help keep the heat out.

Janet was listing to the right side and started to curl up into a fetal position. We kept Janet in bed for safety and comfort measures. I wondered if husband and wife would die within days of each other. But that would not be the case! Several days after this event, Janet's symptoms plateaued. She ate baby food and then soft fruit. Her bowels became active again after an enema, and she continued with oxygen use 24/7 to maintain O2 sats for comfort levels.

A few weeks later, Laura got Covid, and Janet also tested positive. She rallied through this with nebulizers and Mucinex, as her symptoms were mild cough and congestion. She went back to her baseline eating of pureed foods and oxygen was only as needed. Six weeks into the Foley catheter placement, UTI symptoms developed with Purple Urine Bag Syndrome (PUBS). A very pungent odor was present, so Laura requested a round of antibiotics.

PUBS is an unusual demonstration in patients with indwelling Foley catheters. Underlying urinary tract infections are the most common cause. The urine is usually a dark brown color. However, interaction with the plastic bag and tubing turns them into a bright purple. The discoloration of the bag characterizes the presence of an infection.

Common risk factors are female sex, dementia diagnosis, chronic indwelling Foley catheters, and chronic constipation.[11] Janet checked off all the risk factors. Laura and I decided to remove the catheter since Janet had a strong history of UTIs, and this intervention would be counterintuitive. Switching to tabbed briefs proved better for her plan of care moving forward.

Interestingly, the stage three pressure injury on her heel completely closed over. That is not something you usually see happen with all the other dynamics Janet had been experiencing in the previous six weeks.

In the months that followed, Janet had more events. She experienced an upper respiratory infection, which resolved with Mucinex, nebulizers, and Tylenol. I didn't think she would pull through as the altered lung sounds were present for the perfect storm. Then, dark discoloration started to develop on the big toe and spread to each toe of the right foot. Dry gangrene had set in.

Intermittent low-grade fevers occurred and were managed with Tylenol. We painted the toes with betadine daily to keep them dry. Mindfulness was practiced with intention as bed care was performed. Fully expecting autoamputation to happen at any time, it did not occur. Every couple of days, Laura observed Janet's legs moving back and forth like riding a bicycle, indicating that enemas were necessary as Janet could not evacuate. The restless leg activity ceased once the enema provided relief.

I wondered how long Janet would live. Her quality of life was nothing like it used to be. Apparently, this was weighing heavy on my heart as I woke up one night with these words so clearly speaking to my spiritual soul:

---

[11] Hindawi, "Title of the Article," https://www.hindawi.com/journals/dm/2017/9131872/.

"It has been nine decades, six years, and three months now. Right around the corner, I see glimpses of my future. Will my daughter be able to let me go?

My lungs are full. My breathing is not good. My toes have no circulation. I want to detach from my physical body, this shell. My soul and my spirit are ready to take flight.

I am fed several times a day and sometimes awoken to eat. I opt for sleep some days, but it is so heavy on me that I don't want to open my eyes. My quality of life has been resigned to the four walls of this bed. I cannot go anywhere. I am trapped and want to be set free.

Over the past several months, with the ups and downs that my body has gone through, I'm just simply trying to die little by little. She has asked for antibiotics several times to keep me going. This time, she has not asked for antibiotics to try and treat what is ailing my lungs. Maybe she is ready to let me go, just maybe.

I know the love that Laura has for me is unconditional and everlasting. The devotion of how she has cared for me is beyond reproach. I know I will see her again.

I am curling up in the fetal position, getting more contracted with every passing day. I am preparing to leave this world in a similar way to how I entered this world. I was connected to my mom at that time. Now, my daughter is connected to me. When will the cord be cut?"

One night, a few hours after baby food was given, Janet went into a semi-responsive state and couldn't swallow anymore. The active dying process had begun.

Laura's routine was disrupted when she no longer had to prepare three meals a day and give medications at the scheduled times. The focus was no longer on the schedule but rather on giving mouth care, turning and repositioning for comfort, and administering Tylenol suppositories. Laura knew her mom could still hear and process, on some level, the words she shared with her. Laura told her, "Mom, I want you to know that you were never a burden to me." She told her with sincerity, "You know you raised me, and I still love you. You must have done something right!" Janet acknowledged with a smile and a chuckle. Yes, our loved ones hear everything you say to them, even when you think they can't hear.

Four days into the active dying process, Laura's soul knew Janet was starting to transition. She said she switched gears that day, and everything she did moving forward was to help her mom pass peacefully. The on-call nurse came to visit, and Janet's breathing was becoming more labored at 36 breaths per minute, so 0.5 ml of morphine and 0.1 ml of Ativan were given by mouth. It took about 30 minutes for her to relax.

Later, Laura climbed into bed with her sweet mom and cuddled with her, knowing it was the last time she would hold this beautiful woman who brought her into the world. Janet only needed one more dose of meds to help with the respiratory effort to stay calm. That evening, Laura just felt like she needed to be in the room with her. She was sitting there and started to get chest pain and experience anxiety.

Laura told me, "I got up and walked to the kitchen, sat down, and kept looking at her and checking in. And then her eyes went wide open. After this, the whole left side of her neck was pulsating. Then the fish out of water breathing began." Janet transitioned to the next realm peacefully a few minutes later. Laura called her sister Ann and said, "This is the call."

The next day, Laura gathered items for the Durable Medical Equipment company to pick up. She saw on the bedside table the journal where she had meticulously written all of the daily care, medications administered, and status of meals and elimination so thoroughly. She opened it up and flipped to the last page. There were no pages left to document. Janet had finished the final chapter of her book, her 96 years well written and full of love.

Hospice Highlights

- It is imperative to build trust with your patient and caregiver at the start of care. Do not wait until two to three weeks in to address these essential issues. If you wait too long, you are missing a critical window in teaching necessary symptom management.
- Educate, Encourage, and Empower (the 3 E's) patient and caregiver on morphine use for air hunger/discomfort. Given in small doses frequently can be more beneficial than larger breakthrough doses spread apart. Ativan is highly complementary for this symptom as well.
- Symptoms of decline with dementia usually include infections such as UTI, URI, and skin.
- Dry Gangrene: clean and keep dry with betadine daily.
- Evaluate the need for and teach the purpose of antibiotics in end-of-life care. There are positives and negatives.
- Carry extra admit packets in your car.

Source

11) Hindawi. "Title of the Article." htttps://www.hindawi.com/journals/dm/2017/9131872/.

PATIENCE

My first meeting with Camellia was an unexpected delight in so many areas. Talk about an independent, outgoing, vibrant, and organized Alaskan woman who knew how to engage your time and attention! Her ability to participate in interactive conversations from day one was a treat to this nurse. I felt like I was her lifelong friend from the very beginning.

It is so unusual to get to know people of this high caliber who possess such a zest for life and who will be open and honest at the start of care. Camellia had just been diagnosed with multiple myeloma. She made it crystal clear to me that there would be NO treatment for this cancer, and she would live as long as God wanted her to. *It was as simple as that!*

Multiple Myeloma affects approximately 7 per 100,000 annually in the U.S. It is a type of cancer that affects plasma cells. Plasma cells are a part of the immune system that make antibodies to help fight off infections. It is difficult to diagnose multiple myeloma as its symptoms often get attributed to other ailments. Symptoms include general back pain, fatigue, nausea, poor appetite, constipation, and excessive thirst.[12]

---

[12] MyMyelomaTeam, "How Does Myeloma Spread Through the Body," https://www.mymyelomateam.com/resources/how-does-myeloma-spread-through-the-body#Common%20Sites%20For%20Multiple%20Myeloma.

Most often, multiple myeloma is diagnosed at the time of metastasis due to the difficulty in diagnosing early on. The cells grow slowly and attack the bones, including the spine, ribs, long bones, and pelvis. Extramedullary lesions can be found in the soft tissue next to the bones.[13] Less often, lesions are found in the skin, liver, central nervous system, or kidneys.[14]

Camellia lived by herself in an adorable little cottage in town. Her favorite pastime was loving on her indoor plants year-round and being outside for the midnight sun's demonstration of fast-growing beauty for our short Alaskan summers. We get to enjoy plants and flowers from June 1st until early September. Sometimes, we can make it until mid-September or until the first frost visits us.

Her walkway was lined with multiple perennials that do well in Alaskan soil. The patterns of Hosta's, Lobelia, and Primrose decorated her cottage like needlework. Her daughter had to help her with the weeding and keeping everything groomed well. The flowers were beautiful adornments that accented her home like a portrait.

If we admit a patient to hospice who lives alone, we make sure there is a plan for when the patient will need caregiving assistance 24/7. This was a lesson we learned the hard way over the years. Talking with the adult children about the power of attorney on admission is imperative. Everyone needs to be on the same page. We are not yet blessed with a hospice house where patients can go for end of life care if they don't have support. Maybe someday we will have this in Alaska. But I knew we were in good hands with Camellia's family as several adult children were on standby to help with her care, and one child was a part of our medical community.

Our visits were filled with snacks at the kitchen table and sharing stories about her life and a bit of mine. Of course, we started with the necessities of vital signs, head-to-toe assessment, and pain

---

[13] MyMyelomaTeam, "How Does Myeloma Spread Through the Body," https://www.mymyelomateam.com/resources/how-does-myeloma-spread-through-the-body#Common%20Sites%20For%20Multiple%20Myeloma.

[14] Mayo Clinic, "Multiple Myeloma: Symptoms and Causes," https://www.mayoclinic.org/diseases-conditions/multiple-myeloma/symptoms-causes/syc-20353378#!#Overview.

check-in. Then we proceeded to what really mattered to her, which was her life review.

She told me of decades of hardships and joys and how regrets turned into peace as her faith became deeply rooted in her life. She had given up drinking years prior, and one of her big concerns was that she didn't want to become addicted to narcotics for pain control. I listened intently to her concerns. We reviewed musical selections that I would text her before the visit, and she could download them to her iPad to listen to while I was there.

This is what I love about being a hospice nurse. We are privileged to participate in the psychosocial, spiritual, and emotional elements with those we care for. It's not just about providing skilled service and then leaving. A connection builds and develops when a patient comes on to service months before passing. We are allowed time to become part of the story of their lives and be a sojourner with them as they prepare their spirit for what is coming next.

Camellia had lost 13 pounds over the past six months. She really enjoyed eating healthy whole foods and making protein and fruit smoothies in the morning. She pushed herself to eat good food and drink at least two liters of water per day.

Her pain initially presented in her neck and right dislocated shoulder, which was wrapped in a sling. We started with Lidocaine patches 4 %, 12 hours on and 12 hours off, and began discussing narcotics and their purpose with terminal cancer. Camellia wanted to hold off on the narcotics as long as possible. She was fearful of the addiction potential. Explaining the difference between psychological addiction and physical dependence is a common theme with many hospice patients.

Taking things slowly and week by week is important as trust is built between nurse and patient. A new sling arrived for her shoulder, which fit better, so we were able to stop the Lidocaine patches to the neck for the time being. Then, the right elbow started to hurt, so we applied a Lidocaine patch to that area.

Camellia started to have some very high blood pressure readings, including 190/90. She would get lightheaded, and everything would turn dark when she stood up. Her pain level was, on average, a 2/10, so it was not pain-oriented. It was not Orthostatic hypertension, also known as postural hypertension, as the high blood pressure readings did not occur abruptly when she moved into an upright position. Every reading was very similar, whether she was sitting, lying, or standing.

The medical director started her on Norvasc 5 mg, increasing to 10 mg at night. Camellia was at very high risk for falls and breaking bones. Her son, who worked during the day, stayed with her at night, while her daughter, who lived close by, was out of town for the next ten days. Then nausea presented, and she was amenable to starting a Scopolamine patch, which helped this symptom. She especially liked that it was changed out every three days.

The blood pressure issues were managed well, but the pain in the neck returned. Camellia was open to trying a muscle relaxer, so I gave her 5 mg. This made her too relaxed, and she positioned her right arm in the wrong way, causing even more pain. We stopped the Flexeril.

Almost every week, we added a new medication. She liked the idea of ibuprofen three times a day for bone pain, so we gave that a try. After a couple of days of it not being very effective, she was ready to try Norco, but only half a tab. Within a day, she was up to 3 ½ tabs of Norco 5/325 mg.

Camellia had been on service for two months and was ready for better pain control. She was also ready for the hospital bed and air mattress. She used a wedge pillow for her feet and made a cozy nest with her set up in her room, which helped with her bone pain. The ease of pressing buttons to help one get in and out of bed cannot be underestimated.

The medical director made a home visit per Camellia's daughter's request to assess how she was doing. He determined the blood pressure issue was positional vertigo and taught her eye exercises to alleviate the dizziness. He also wrapped her right shoulder/arm in the sling in a unique way to reduce the pain levels.

Camellia loved her CNA, who came several times per week to help with her personal care and showers. The social worker assisted one of her daughters with the long-term care insurance paperwork to help her get paid for personal care assistant work. This was a better plan than Camellia going to an assisted living facility. Camellia also enjoyed the Chaplain's routine visits. It was beautiful to see a patient

PATIENCE

so receptive to everyone on the team. She was walking through her journey with grace, gratitude, and patience.

The pain in her bones spread to the hips and ribs. Her mobility was decreasing noticeably with every visit. The plan was for one of her daughters to move in with her within the next week. Camellia worried about too much Tylenol in the Norco, so the medical director changed it to oxycodone.

Constipation increased, so a combination of Senna S and Sorbitol was used. I had to give suppositories and enemas to get things moving. She didn't realize it had been several days since a bowel movement. Her appetite was declining rapidly, and confusion started.

She was ready to try liquid morphine to get faster pain relief. Her pain reduced from a 6 to a 3/10 within 20 minutes. Morphine replaced the oxycodone tablets. Suddenly, jaundice appeared. She was almost bedbound but still managed to get to the bedside commode. We also implemented the Nicotine patch as she was no longer able to go outside to smoke.

Camillia's daughter had arrived, and she was so happy. It had been two decades since all of her children were together with her. The children honored her request to move the hospital bed out to the living room so Camillia could be with all of her beautiful plants. Over the next week, she enjoyed everyone being under one roof and sharing stories.

One unique pet also came to visit. A pet duck of one of the grandkids, who was very well-behaved and wore a little diaper. He would prance around to different family members and snuggle just like a little dog.

The week before she became bed-bound, she told me I could have a few of her Maranta Leucon Eura prayer plant clippings to grow some roots. Then, I would have my own plant as a beautiful reminder of our friendship. I took a few clippings home and placed them in a clear quart-sized jar.

I told Camellia I didn't have any roots springing forth yet in the water and wondered if it would ever happen. Her pale blue eyes turned, and she looked at me from her transient state of peace. She said, "Esther, it's only been ten days. Be patient."

How did she remember it had only been ten days? I thought it was fascinating that she could keep track of this detail while she was doing the intense inner work of processing and preparing for her departure. But somehow, Camellia still understood the passage of time.

She embraced having all her family tending to her needs and the activity that enveloped her once "private" home. Her eyes conveyed such an astonishing tranquility and calm look that it was hard to put into words. I will never forget that special moment as Camellia taught me so many beautiful things while I cared for her. She had come to know that I struggled with the fruit of being patient, and she encouraged me to embrace this.

It was time for a Foley catheter as we could not roll and turn her easily due to the dislocated shoulder in the sling for brief changes. Camillia wanted to wear oxygen for comfort, and at four liters, saturation would rise to 91%. The family was open to end-of-life teaching and comfort measures, which was truly heartwarming. We started a Fentanyl patch at 25 mcg for long-acting control and soon doubled to 50 mcg. Camellia went into a nonresponsive state; her oxygen levels gently titrated down, and she passed peacefully with all of her children present.

I relished every visit and getting to know Camellia over the five months she was on service. You know how they say it's important to talk to your plants? The week I wrote Camellia's story, I talked to my prayer plant and said it was time to write her story. Over the next two weeks, four new stems started to grow. That has never happened with this plant! My prayer plant is lush and thriving to this day.

I hope I understand a little of what she encouraged me to do, to have patience. Camellia was the master gardener! She planted the seed of endurance from her garden into me when I needed it the most. This came to be a few years later during my extended, painful leg recovery.

PATIENCE

> **Hospice Highlights**
>
> - Acknowledge and embrace what your patients give to you. It isn't a one-way street.
> - Recognize if there is an addiction history and empower your patient to make decisions when they are ready for more effective pain management.

Source

12) MyMyelomaTeam. "How Does Myeloma Spread Through the Body." https://www.mymyelomateam.com/resources/how-does-myeloma-spread-through-the-body#Common%20Sites%20For%20Multiple%20Myeloma.
13) MyMyelomaTeam. "How Does Myeloma Spread Through the Body." https://www.mymyelomateam.com/resources/how-does-myeloma-spread-through-the-body#Common%20Sites%20For%20Multiple%20Myeloma.
14) Mayo Clinic. "Multiple Myeloma: Symptoms and Causes." https://www.mayoclinic.org/diseases-conditions/multiple-myeloma/symptoms-causes/syc-20353378#!#Overview.

SPEED IT UP

At age 86, Linda had been living on her cattle ranch in the "lower 48" for 16 years after her husband passed away. She was involved in her circle of activities with friends and church. She kept up with managing the house as best she could until her cardiac diagnosis began to advance into the final stages.

She had a stroke in the springtime, which left her with right-sided weakness and residual tingling. She also had an abdominal aortic aneurism that was leaking and needed to be repaired. They fixed it, but then she subsequently became weaker and needed more care with all of her daily living activities.

In October, her daughter, Sue, flew her up to Alaska to live with her and her husband. There were grandchildren and great-grandchildren ready to give Linda a new circle of life in the final months that she would journey. Later that month, several aortic stents were placed, which seemed successful. But then, Linda had orthostatic blood pressure issues after the stents, and her heart would stop and then start again. She needed beta-blockers, but the pacemaker needed to be placed first.

After the pacemaker insertion, she went to cardiac rehab at a skilled facility. The goal was to gain independence with using the bathroom and to be able to climb some stairs, but Linda was not making any improvements. She wasn't willing to do the exercises.

According to Sue, Linda had to want it. Her mom had the type of personality that wanted things to come easily in life. Sue did not want her relationship with her mom to be one of nagging her to keep pushing for rehab if she wasn't willing to do so.

Of course, all of this transpired during a surge of Covid, and Linda was ready to come home for Christmas. She started on home health services for physical therapy and occupational therapy to no avail. The cardiologist said nothing was working properly. The pacemaker was not pacing as it should, and medications were not helping improve her quality of life.

It was time for the transition to hospice care a few days after Christmas. Linda was agreeable and ready. In the months that followed, Sue was the primary caregiver. Linda wouldn't allow her son-in-law to help much with transfers and care. She could somewhat shuffle with weak ambulation steps to help. More often though, she would have issues with passing out on the commode. Sue would help her get revived by having her sit on the commode and hold her feet up until her blood pressure rose again. The pain of sitting on the commode would help raise the blood pressure as well.

It was very taxing for Sue to do all the personal care and was emotionally exhausting. Due to the discomfort, Linda didn't want Sue to use the safety belt for transfers. Inevitably, one day, they both went to the ground with the transfer. At this point, Linda became bedbound, and a whole other level of care began. A respite stay was provided for Linda, and Sue was able to enjoy a much-needed break for five days.

Sue was very active in her retired life, helping with caring for her grandchildren and enjoying many hobbies and activities with her family. Linda was financially prepared for this stage in life and decided it was time to move into an assisted living facility. She had previously been on the waitlist for the independent side, so it was a smooth transition. When she was ready to move, there was an opening on the ALF side with nursing care.

I asked Sue months later how she reconciled with the feelings of her mom leaving her home and moving into assisted living. She had me laughing when she told me she was a "recovering Catholic" because, with every decision she made, considerable *guilt* was associated with it. She was pragmatic about the decision, and her husband was very supportive.

When I met Linda for the first time (4 months on service), it was springtime in Alaska, and I was on call. Linda was still at Sue's home. Her pain was increasing, and the liquid morphine taste was undesirable and difficult to get down, so a low-dose Fentanyl patch was ordered. I picked up the medication and brought it with me to the visit. Linda's pain areas were two-fold, with chest pain and pain associated with the skin breakdown that began in the sacral area three weeks after admission. She was taking in small amounts of fluid, not eating much, and sleeping more.

Appearing to be making progress in the *Gone From My Sight* book symptoms of weeks prognosis; we talked about symptoms and what she may or may not go through with her cardiac diagnosis. Linda begged for one more week to stay with Sue before she had to go to the assisted living facility. She was ready to stop taking all her cardiac medications and did so.

Linda asked to have her pacemaker turned "off." A call was put into the cardiologist group, and they refused because it was considered *Euthanasia*. The belief being that the pacemaker was keeping her alive, and turning it off would be, in essence, giving someone a death sentence.

This didn't make any sense to me. How was this any different than someone being on a ventilator and the patient deciding to come off of this "machine" but can't with a device that was implanted? I explained to Linda and Sue exactly what the cardiologist group told me. She was frustrated with their decision.

The next week, I took over as her case manager when she moved into the ALF in my patient area. Linda chose to remain in bed and did not want to interact with the other residents. She was quite content to be in her room. She enjoyed watching the Hallmark channels and crocheting. The priest and volunteers from the church routinely came to visit, which she looked forward to. Her family and daughter would visit regularly to brighten her day.

Symptom issues arose with constipation. We started with suppositories and oral stool softeners. Eventually, we had to proceed to enemas twice weekly and then three times weekly to ensure a balanced routine. This would help avoid weekend on-call visits for symptom management that should be regulated during the week. Linda had a unique presentation with her lower colon and many inverted loops in the lower GI tract. The procedure of enemas usually required digital removal, which she didn't have the strength to eliminate.

As the months progressed, Linda continued to lose weight and muscle mass. Since we couldn't weigh her in bed, we kept track of the MAC, mid-arm circumference measurement. As her heart muscle continued to deteriorate, the chest pain would increase at times. She was more willing to take the liquid morphine on a schedule now, along with the Fentanyl dose, which slowly increased every few months in dosage. Lorazepam didn't work as it caused hallucinations, so that was listed as an allergy/sensitivity. We stuck with Haldol, as needed for anxiety, and this helped nausea symptoms also.

Five months into Linda being on service, the weight loss was very noticeable. The liquid morphine was causing hallucinations as it would absorb into her bloodstream faster. The medical director ordered Morphine Sulfate immediate-release tablets three times per day to help with breakthrough pain.

In August, three months after starting the MSIR tabs, Linda called the family in and said it was her time to go, and she wanted to say goodbye. She was experiencing 20-second periods of apnea, and her heart rate was very irregular when sleeping heavily. Three days later, she pulled out of the episode and went back to her baseline. I didn't think anything of it because I've seen patients experience active dying symptoms, then snap back out and plateau. We had been riding the slow-moving roller coaster of ups and downs for many months.

One month later, during a normal visit, Linda wanted help with her mouth care. I helped take her partial denture out and was looking for her container to place it in for cleaning. I found it, and something rattled when I picked it up. I asked Linda what the rattling was, and she tried to grab the box out of my hands!

I was completely shocked to find 13 MSIR tabs stockpiled. I asked her why, and was just completely flabbergasted. Sue was just as shocked as I was at how she was able to trick the staff and hide the pills. Linda had been non-compliant with her stool softeners, so trying to put her on an antidepressant would have been to no avail. At this point, we discontinued the MSIR tablets, and the Fentanyl patch was increased for pain control. If she needed a dose of liquid morphine for breakthrough pain, it was available.

Upon further discussion, Linda revealed that she had tried this a month prior when she called the family in to say goodbye and had the "episode" that she had pulled out of. Needless to say, I had my radar up now and was more in tune with situations like this when the patient called the family in to say goodbye and then started the active symptoms of dying.

It was February now, and Linda had made it to her 88th birthday! She would ask from time to time why it took so long to die. I would explain to her that her body had made many changes with losing weight, pressure injury in her sacral area, and her heart was getting weaker overall. But maybe God had more plans for her, with interaction and time with her family, and it wasn't her time quite yet.

She would try and keep busy with crocheting blankets, but her depression was still underlying. She looked forward to the priest visits and phone calls from her priest back home. A common theme in our talks was that she believed the pills were keeping her alive. She was only on a few stool softeners and a stomach acid pill; that was it. I explained that it was nutrition keeping her alive: food and liquids. I described how, as people get closer to their bodies shutting down, the food intake naturally declined to no intake at all, and death would usually occur within ten days.

By mid-April, she said she was ready to stop eating and drinking and let go of the feeling that she had *to push herself to do so*. I encouraged her that we would keep her comfortable. She stopped eating most foods, ate just a few bites, and drank apple juice. Later, she went down to just green sponges dipped in apple juice to keep her mouth moist.

One Friday morning, I walked into her apartment with a nurse I was training. We waited in the living room, witnessing Linda's extremely engaging conversation with multiple people. People who weren't there. She was seeing people in the room as she looked upwards and to the corner, pointing and engaging. It was very clear she was starting to *transition* as she engaged in the next spiritual realm with such vitality and discussion. Finally, she finished her conversation and motioned with her hands for us to come into her room. Her blood pressure was 140/90, pulse at 75, respirations at 14, and O2 saturation at 97% with 20-second periods of apnea. We documented the information and left.

Three hours later, I received a frantic call from Sue that Linda had Fixodent stuck in her mouth and nose. Her granddaughter had come to visit and found her like this. Linda had tried to end her life by blocking her airways. I diverted from a visit to head back to the ALF.

Upon arrival, she was in a deep, unarousable sleep. We used green sponges and coconut oil to remove the material from her nose and mouth. After 40 minutes of working to remove the sticky substance, it loosened up. She was placed on a routine schedule with Haldol liquid to keep her calm. *Everything but a call light was removed from her bedside.*

Full side rails were up on both sides of the hospital bed. We placed a mattress on the floor next to the bed for safety and put signs on the wall for further safety reminders for staff. Sue said that later on, she wanted the easy way out and a quick fix. But who would have thought of Fixodent? She was placed on daily nursing visits, as we like to do when patients are in their last week or so, as symptoms can change daily, and med management and support are more intensive.

That Saturday, Sue was at her bedside watching her sleep. Linda's eyes flared open, and she looked at Sue and started yelling, "Call him, Call him!" She lifted her right arm, the weak side she could *never* lift, and said it again. She was mad! Sue said, "I'll take care of it." And then it was ok.

Then she yelled, "I don't love you; I hate you," looking right at Sue. Gradually, she started to calm down. This was the beginning of her surge of energy. She went back to sleep. Who knows what this stark and angry conversation was about? Undoubtedly, these two had a close bond as mother and daughter. Linda had never talked to Sue like this before.

Even though she was apprehensive after the harsh words on Saturday, Sunday was Mother's Day, and Sue said the Catholic guilt made her visit. The nursing staff said Linda was awake, and they had been talking with her. It was hard for her to talk as her voice was weaker. Linda wanted to give her son a "reply" (her words were not always making sense). He was a joy in her life, and they talked with him on the phone.

SPEED IT UP

She had an awareness of what was happening. She seemed to be happy, excited, and accepting of the process. Linda said, "Since I'm on my way... can I have something to drink now?" She sipped apple juice and started choking. She stated, "Well, I won't do that again!"

Sue said it was like she had a resolution and resolve about her. She knew she had made progress on the *path* and was ready. Sunday, the surge was over. Linda had no recollection of the Fixodent incident the day prior.

On Monday, when I came to visit, Kennedy's ulcer showed up in the mid-spine, and the sacral wound was deteriorating even further. Linda couldn't talk, but she knew the routine and tried to use her hand to hold the bedrail when we turned her. We applied the Scopolamine patch to prepare for secretions to occur, which I anticipated with a cardiac diagnosis, but this didn't happen.

By Wednesday, she was in a deep sleep, and we padded up the sacral area with multiple dressings for absorption. Sue did not like seeing this part of the care. However, she wanted to be a part of helping and handed me the dressings. Her analogy of what she saw was like a "zombie salmon" when they are at the end of life, and their bodies start to disintegrate and fall apart. I knew that was very difficult for her to do and see, but she needed to.

Linda's beginning weight was 131 pounds, and in her last week of life, I estimated that she was 85 pounds. Her final dosage of Fentanyl patch reached 125 mcg. Even though she didn't have much muscle mass, it did work for her in achieving optimal pain management.

Linda chose to leave this earth on a holiday of sorts, Friday the 13th. She found peace that final week and surrendered to the process. Even though she tried to speed that course up a few times, the natural progression of her cardiac illness played out over 17 very long months. The biggest shock to Sue in all of this was how slow and measured her decline was and the attempt Linda made with the pills and Fixodent to end things more quickly.

Linda taught me many valuable lessons as I cared for her for that year. Even though we may want to leave before our time, this realm is out of our control. There is an intrinsic purpose in our humanity, and we will never know the impact we have on those we love the most. What we offer from our spirit and soul affects those around us. Someday, all will be revealed, and we will understand why our remarkable journey carried out the path it was uniquely designed to take.

HOSPICE HIGHLIGHTS

- Cardiac decline symptoms may include skin breakdown, weight loss, chest pain, dizziness, and upper respiratory infections.
- Explore the symptoms of depression and ask if self-harm is in the patient's thought process; adjust the plan of care moving forward.
- Be on alert if the patient suddenly demonstrates an active dying process.

CULTURAL DIVERSITIES

I would like to preface the following stories with background amongst the Native American (NA) population regarding death and dying. The discussion includes the death taboo perception from a historical observation. According to Merriam-Webster, taboo is defined as a social or religious custom prohibiting or forbidding discussion of a particular practice or unfriendly association with a particular person, place, or thing.

The majority of NAs who hold true to their ancestral values believe in the Creator, Great Spirit, or God, which governs all living creatures equally, including humans. Death is understood as part of the natural life cycle. There are two types of spirits: physical and spiritual. While death means the physical body has died, the spiritual one continues by crossing over to the spiritual realm. Death is a continuum, not the end of all life. Because of this, death should not be feared. It is the Creator's obligation to govern each creature's purpose. Discussion of death and dying can be considered irreverence towards the Creator.[15]

In light of this awareness, the hospice nurse needs a full understanding of these concepts when working with NAs: 1) death is not

---

[15] Jennifer R. Gray and Barbara S. Thomas, "Native American Death Taboo: Implications for Health Care Providers," https://www.researchgate.net/publication/298726050_Native_American_DeathTaboo_Implications_for_Health_Care_Providers.

in human control but in the Creator's realm to determine, 2) calming evil spirits requires silence to decrease harm, and 3) countenance of death may initiate another demise due to the *power of words*.

Based on these cultural perceptions, hospice nurses must present themselves in a delicate manner and with an empathetic approach. As communication is exchanged with the family, elders, and patient, trust can be built over time. Time may not be on our side with late referrals to hospice, a few weeks before the dying process begins.

A critical factor to identify at the start of care is what level of medical actions and medications the patient will be comfortable with. Is it a part of the Creator's will or not? They may not place a high value on understanding and knowing all the information that is present.[16] This is a dilemma for the hospice nurse as we are supposed to teach and educate on every visit, preparing the patient for the impending transition. Often, the valued relationship between patient and doctor plays an important role in determining the medications allowed and details of the plan of care implemented.

Several gentle encouragements and discussions on subject matters may need to transpire due to an indirect communication style. Explaining why a comfort pack of emergency medications needs to be in the home on day one and the purpose of a 'do not resuscitate' order is of great importance; however, it may take multiple conversations over several visits to accomplish.

While these stories highlight cultural sensitivity for NAs, it is noteworthy to say understanding every patient's individual culture is critical.

---

[16] Jennifer R. Gray and Barbara S. Thomas, "Native American Death Taboo: Implications for Health Care Providers," https://www.researchgate.net/publication/298726050_Native_American_DeathTaboo_Implications_for_Health_Care_Providers.

Source

15) Gray, Jennifer R., and Barbara S. Thomas. "Native American Death Taboo: Implications for Health Care Providers." https://www.researchgate.net/publication/298726050_Native_American_DeathTaboo_Implications_for_Health_Care_Providers.
16) Gray, Jennifer R., and Barbara S. Thomas. "Native American Death Taboo: Implications for Health Care Providers." https://www.researchgate.net/publication/298726050_Native_American_DeathTaboo_Implications_for_Health_Care_Providers.

THE DOCTORS ROLE

I met William on his first day as I did his start-of-care intake. William was 69 years old. He had been sent home from the ER five days prior with a diagnosis of Covid and was told, "You are fine, and the x-ray of your lungs is good," even though he was very short of breath. His wife Sarah called their primary physician to explain what happened at the ER and that they needed more help and care.

William's lungs presented with mild respiratory distress, a cough, and saturating at 93% on room air. His lung sounds included rhonchi and wheezing. He had completed a telehealth visit with his primary provider four days after the ER visit, and this is when we received the order to initiate hospice care. His primary diagnosis was end-stage Parkinson's disease. William was an Alaskan native, and his wife was indigenous. The relationship these two had with their primary physician had been long-standing for 15 years plus, with unequivocal trust.

William's comorbidity list included a history of deep vein thrombosis for which he wore compression stockings daily and anxiety disorder with a touch of OCD. He was over six feet tall and had lost over 35 pounds in the past year. William was mobile with his walker and stand-by assist. He moved very deliberately and at a slow pace.

But over the past year, William had fallen five times, luckily with no injuries. Every time, Sarah had to call family to help get him off the floor. In two incidences, she called 911 because he was choking on his food, and she had to perform the Heimlich maneuver. William did not like blended or pureed foods. He was still eating solid foods.

At the time of admission, William absolutely did not want to sign the POLST form (do not resuscitate). He made it very clear that he did not want to go back to the hospital ever again and wanted to stay at home and be kept comfortable. Sarah and William had been married for 40 years. Sarah struggled with anxiety, also. I thought it best to table the POLST discussion for later.

The equipment of the bedside table, oxygen, and nebulizer machine arrived later that afternoon after I had left on admission day. Everyone was reluctant to put the oxygen on to see if it would help William. The next day, during my follow-up visit, William's saturation levels increased to 95 on room air. However, the cough had gotten worse. Sarah and his sister Maureen were up most of the night, tending to his needs but not using any of the tools yet.

I had to negotiate with William, "Let's give the oxygen and nebulizer a try and see if you feel any better." He agreed, and after each was implemented, he felt some relief. Then, I asked if he would try a tiny dose of liquid morphine. After explaining how it helped relax the respiratory effort, he agreed to dry a dose of 0.1 ml (2 mg). It worked, and he was relieved it didn't have any side effects.

William was rather stoic and did not like medications in general. He was only on a few prescriptions for Parkinson's symptoms and one to prevent further blood clots. Upon further discussion of his daily routine, Sarah explained she was feeding William in bed at a 30-degree angle.

We did some teaching about keeping him up to a 90-degree angle propped with pillows since he was in his own bed, not the hospital bed. This would help keep him from choking again or aspirating. Sarah was receptive to the teaching and said she would start doing this.

In ten days on service, William reduced the nebulizer treatments to two times a day as his lung sounds improved, but a small lingering cough was still present. William's goal was to make it to the dining area three times a week for interaction and meal time. Over the next few months, William's energy levels slowly declined, and he could not make it to the dining room. The nebulizers continued, usually once per day. He was aspirating every so often, with mild rhonchi sounds present and oxygen saturation levels of around 91% on room air.

Two months had gone by, and William presented with skin breakdown on his inner buttocks. It had the appearance of shearing and feathered skin. It progressed from stage one to two, closed over, and then opened up again. How often William agreed to reposition in the bed influenced his skin condition. Sarah did the wound care, applying Calazime when redness was present, and when it opened up, she applied a foam dressing for absorption.

William had bouts with loose stools, usually because of what he ate. One day, he had too much chocolate. Sarah thought it was good for his spirits to allow him to choose his foods as so many decisions were being taken away from him. Usually, the bowel regimen would be three times a week. Due to the nature of Parkinson's and losing muscle control for evacuation, enemas oftentimes had to be instituted. Stool softeners were not really in his protocol, as he would rather eat fruit. But incontinence was occurring more often.

William had a good setup around his "own" bed with hand bars on the walls, a partial half rail on the side of the bed, and devices for him to hold. The stiffness and rigidity over his entire body were increasing. He was maxed on the Parkinson's medications. Still, he did not want to start any new prescription to help, such as a muscle relaxer. Being as alert as possible was of great importance to him. He did not like the feeling of the pillows around his body to help tilt him side to side to get pressure off of his tailbone. He said it made him feel 'claustrophobic.'

As often occurs as this disease progresses, the strength decreases. William fell as he was holding on to a rail attached to his bed while getting up. He landed on his right arm, which displayed a very bright-colored yellow and green hematoma with a decent amount of hard swelling. His range of motion was good, and pain was very low, so it appeared it was not fractured. He was amenable to a compression wrap to get the swelling to go down. This took about one month to resolve; he was also on a blood thinner.

As symptoms advanced, his speech deteriorated. William would try to say a word, but it would take a minute to even speak one word (dysarthria). We would guess what he was trying to say to meet his needs. His hands were too weak to communicate with writing. It was fascinating to see how some days were better, and then he would go back down again and stay on that lower rung on the ladder, never advancing upward. He would no longer go to the dining room; his world became his bedroom and bathroom.

It is always important to chart in the negative for hospice patients, as we are to show signs and symptoms of decline. A picture must be painted of the actual symptoms of decline, however minor they may seem. With a noncancerous diagnosis, patients can be on service for several years as long as the decline is legitimate and documentation reflects the patient's status.

In regards to the cultural diversities, William made it clear to me on week one that he was 'Not that into a lot of medications.' He was willing to do the nebulizer treatments to help his lungs improve. He wanted me to get rid of the oxygen after the first week, but I convinced him it should stay in the house in time of a crisis.

As your relationship as the hospice nurse grows with your patient, they will slowly come to respect your advice over time. Both William and Sarah were a private couple. They didn't like it when I had a day off and a pool nurse would visit. At times, they would cancel that nurse.

I tried to get our CNA to help with personal care because I wanted more of the hospice team involved, but they refused as they wanted to keep their hired CNA. They also declined chaplain support. I was glad he tried the morphine at least once that first week and conquered some fear and anxiety. This was important in how William's story concluded.

Six months on service, and still, I was at a roadblock on the "Do not resuscitate" issue. I asked William's devoted doctor to make a house call, relying on the valued relationship between the patient and the doctor. He was the only one who could get through to him. It didn't matter how many ways I explained it.

When the doctor visited, he discussed the rationale for the Do Not Resuscitate form, as Williams's overall condition was declining in multiple areas. They discussed what would happen if 911 was called and that he might wind up on life support. Was this what he truly wanted?

The doctor didn't have the actual form during the visit, so I reviewed the sections two visits later. William was comfortable having

Sarah sign off on it since she was his Power of Attorney for healthcare. William's doctor played an invaluable role in his final days. He also convinced William to try the air mattress on top of his own bed to help his skin condition.

Another month went by with no new symptoms. Then, on a Monday, I received a panicked call from Sarah. William was not doing well at all. He would not let her call yesterday when everything started. He was having loose bowel movements, nausea, vomiting, fever, and chills.

When I arrived with my new trainee, we found William in severe respiratory distress, sitting on the bedside commode. He was very pale and ashen, and his feet were mottled. His oxygen levels were 80% on room air, and respirations at 30 per minute.

We got him back to the bed with a gait belt and did a head-to-toe assessment. His abdomen was distended on the left side and extremely hard, and his right side was less firm. He had active bowel sounds in all four quadrants, and his lungs were clear.

His pain level was definitely approaching severe. We gave him a dose of Ativan to help his anxiety and a dose of morphine (the little that was left in the bottle). Sarah had accidentally spilled the majority of the bottle of morphine the night prior. The oxygen was on at five liters. When he rose to the mid-90s saturation levels, we titrated down to two liters.

We called the medical director with the assessment findings, which he said had the appearance of a perforated bowel and the potential for peritonitis. We offered William the option of going to the hospital for treatment or staying at home and being comfortable with medications if he would allow it. We explained that with these symptoms, his transition would be quick within a few days. William clearly expressed his desire to stay at home.

We inserted a Foley catheter, which was a negotiation as well. We explained that having to turn him often for brief changes would be too painful for his abdomen. We ordered the hospital bed, and it arrived at shift change. It took 4 personnel from the nonemergent EMS team to safely move him; he was tall and about 190 pounds. The on-call nurse visited to make sure he was tucked in for the night. The nurse also inserted the Macey catheter for ease of med administration with morphine and Ativan.

Another family member picked up more meds and Fentanyl, so the nurse pre-drew up syringes of each med to make things easier for Sarah and Maureen to administer. Sarah was very tearful and was very blessed to have the support of her sister-in-law, Maureen. Their hired CNA was there as well to help with the care those first few hours.

During my visit the next morning, William could answer a few questions. The pain was under better control. They were giving him medications every four hours. That evening, Sarah called and said his breathing was worse, and he was grunting. The on-call nurse visited and received orders to give 7 ml (140 mg) of morphine over the course of 2 1/2 hours, and the Fentanyl patch was doubled to 100 mcg and 2 mg of Ativan to help with anxiety via the Macey catheter.

William's pain finally calmed down, and he was able to rest. Four hours later, the on-call nurse received the call that William had passed. It was a traumatic experience for Sarah to see as coffee ground emesis occurred in a large volume. Maureen was present and tried to help Sarah in her grief.

I regret not educating and explaining to Sarah the potential for the dramatic ending with the coffee ground emesis. I didn't think she would have taken the information well in advance due to her anxiety levels. Not everyone is a planner with "the-more-information-the-better" motto.

After William died, I sent condolences in a message as Sarah didn't answer the phone. Several days later, I received a call from Maureen, and she had Sarah on the line on speaker phone. Sarah was angry, crying, and grieving heavily. She said she felt abandoned in the final hours, and they shouldn't have been alone while William was dying.

I listened to her cry and be angry and let it all out. Sometimes you have to hold presence over the phone, as we often do in person. Sarah stated she didn't want to live. I asked her if she had a plan to harm herself, and she said no. Maureen said she would not leave her alone. I asked Maureen to please get her to see her medical provider as soon as possible. I also encouraged them to attend our weekly bereavement group that the chaplain hosted. Maureen said she would try to bring her. I notified the chaplain to follow up and offer support.

Grief can be full of a wide variety of emotions, and as the hospice nurse, you may be the recipient of harsh words. The dying process is not always physically peaceful, as the body is weakened when shutting down. I was thankful that the POLST form had been signed one month prior to William's passing, or it may have been more dramatic with EMS involved.

Even though Sarah knew William's spirit had continued to the next realm, this did not bring her comfort as his dramatic and quick departure rattled her to the core. She was not ready for him to leave. There is only so much a hospice nurse can do to prepare for anticipatory grief of the significant other when they struggle to engage in the process. This is where bereavement support and follow-up in the months after the patient dies are important. The potential for processing is available if the family is willing to participate.

Hospice Highlights

- The valued relationship between patient and doctor often plays an important role in determining the medications allowed and details of the plan of care implemented.
- Determine what level of medical actions and medications the patient will be comfortable with.
- The family member will choose when they are ready to begin the grieving process.
- Awareness and respect for cultural and family values are important for how and when you broach sensitive topics.

THE POWER OF WORDS

Ahna, who was 85 years old, had been living with her daughter, Carla, for several years. Her hospice diagnosis was senile degeneration of the brain. Her comorbidity list included protein-calorie malnutrition, type 2 diabetes, chronic kidney disease stage 1-4, and osteoporosis. I was not her case manager, but I offered to help with a few visits as the team struggled to navigate some challenging circumstances.

Ahna was on service for a brief four weeks. Pain was not an issue initially; it was more insomnia, reverse sleep schedules, and agitation. Carla informed us that the agitation (Sundowners symptoms) occurred for six months. Multiple medications were tried in the first few weeks to help Ahna sleep and with the agitation. These included Trazodone with melatonin, Haldol, and Ativan. We tried morphine for the pain.

Along with these symptoms, her nutritional status was dwindling quickly. Her food intake was primarily sips of Ensure. Carla gave her mom the oral tablets crushed, but there was no consistency in the administration of the as-needed meds for agitation and pain management.

Carla was struggling with her mom's disease progression and would say, "She was going to get up again and be ok." Education was given by the case manager from *Gone From My Sight* on the disease process and the purpose of medications to bring comfort during the dying process[17]. However, the information did not appear to be taking hold with the family.

When another family member flew in from the village, she informed us that 'The Elders said she didn't need any morphine.' We began to notice a trend two weeks in that the on-call nurse would be notified to come out at night due to pain. The family would ask her to give the morphine. They didn't say why, but they wanted support.

At the time, our case managers took turns with on-call duties on average, two nights per month, and two weeks of the month we had an on-call nurse. Each person can triage things a little differently. However, it is important to be on the same page with boundaries. On-call visits should be for active dying crises and support, death calls, and other emergencies. When routine calls come in at 5:01 pm asking a nurse to come and give morphine, someone in the family must be identified to be able to give medication.

One night, Carla called because Ahna hadn't voided in 12 hours. When the nurse arrived, she had been incontinent, so she was cleaned and repositioned. The nurse offered a Foley catheter, which the family declined. Putting tubes in to alleviate a symptom would further define where Ahna was in the dying process, and they weren't ready for that.

I offered to make a visit for the case manager to help communicate with the family about Ahna's condition and their hesitancy to give Ahna medication. Ahna had been on service for three weeks, and the case manager thought a Kennedy's ulcer was starting to develop on her coccyx.

When I arrived, both daughters and older grandchildren were present. I did Ahna's assessment but asked if I could give morphine prior as I would have to roll and turn her, and there was wound care to do. They agreed, and I premedicated Ahna. She did well with the care and repositioning. Ahna appeared to be starting to transition to the final stages as she was curling up into the fetal position. I applied the Scopolamine patch for secretions as they were starting to manifest.

---

[17] Barbara Karnes, *Gone From My Sight: The Dying Experience* (Vancouver, WA: Barbara Karnes Books, 1986).

One of the daughters asked if I could fill out her Family Medical Leave paperwork. I agreed because this would be an opportunity to talk about medication management and preparation for what was coming. Before I began the paperwork, I asked if I could review the blue book with the family. I knew this had *already* been done a few times prior, but now was the time to find out where they were in understanding Ahna's imminence.

After checking off all the symptoms for the "weeks" category, I explained that Ahna was now moving into the "days" portion. Both daughters started to cry, and emotions flowed. I listened to their grief and dug deeper into the medication issue. Carla had lost her spouse a few years prior, so it was very difficult to be losing her Mom now. She felt like it was one right after the other, and she hadn't processed losing her spouse.

After listening to the daughters express their sorrow and offering support, I asked Carla if she had concerns about giving morphine to help her mom be comfortable. She reiterated that the elders from the village told her 'That Ahna didn't need morphine.' (Death is not in human control, but in the Creator's realm to determine).

She and her sister felt torn about giving pain medication as their elders told them not to, but seeing their mom in pain was tearing them apart on the inside. I may have been a little brass, but I explained the elders were not here to see what Ahna was experiencing in her dying process. She was having pain and needed help for her body to relax and transcend to the next spiritual realm. Carla told me she was afraid of overdosing her mom with morphine. So, there were two issues underlying the reluctance to give pain medication. They felt more comfortable with the nurses giving the medication.

I asked if they would agree to a low-dose Fentanyl patch placed on her skin to give time-released medication. The nurse could apply it and change it every 72 hours. They agreed, so I asked the medical director to write the order for a 12 mcg patch as Ahna had been receiving morphine for several weeks but only on average one to two times a day. She did have enough in her system to tolerate the Fentanyl patch of 12 mcg. The on-call nurse came out that night, applied the patch, and showed the family how to use the Yonker Suction machine as secretions began.

The next night, Ahna started the fish out of water, breathing, and the family thought she was dying right then. The on-call nurse visited to offer support and gave a dose of morphine to help her breathing relax. The breathing patterns continued to change over the next few days. The following day, the granddaughter was willing to give morphine to help the symptoms as her pulse was up to 140, and her breathing was labored. In the last few days, Ahna had mild apnea 20 seconds long and oxygen levels at 88%. She passed peacefully that night, surrounded by her children and many grandchildren.

Valuable lessons were learned caring for Ahna. Understanding ancestral values was significant as this was the foundation of the Native American population. Finding a way to work with the family members to manage pain and symptoms is crucial while respecting cultural diversity.

Hospice Highlights

- Respect cultural diversities when teaching about the dying process. The two have to find a balance as we are preparing families for the death of their loved ones.
- Utilize transdermal patches for pain management in these types of challenging scenarios.
- On-call nurses establish boundaries and follow protocol for what constitutes the need for on-call visits. Case Managers need to communicate within the same boundaries.
- Bringing in a "fresh" or new nurse for a visit can help open new lines of communication and additional perspectives.

Source

17) Karnes, Barbara. Gone From My Sight: The Dying Experience. Vancouver, WA: Barbara Karnes Books, 1986.

IN SHOCK

Ivan's daughter Alena greeted me at the front door on my first visit. Alena was very pleasant and fluent in English. She was visiting from out of state. She would be one of the interpreters for her dad, Ivan, and her mom, Katya. Both parents only spoke Russian.

Ivan and Katya lived in Sasha's home. She was the oldest daughter and participated in this first visit via phone while on a break from work. Sasha wanted me to review the lab results from the day before Ivan was admitted to Hospice. We went over the results, and nothing was significantly notable.

Part of the discussion on the day after admission to hospice was reviewing the magnitude of Ivan's diagnosis. This was a very rare cancer, and when it spread this quickly, comfort measures were the only option. They inquired about going to Seattle for surgical interventions, but the oncologist explained that this was not a possibility.

They were processing and grieving so heavily. It was important to allow space and time for this to occur. We had many steps to walk through quickly, and the family needed time to vent during day one. I was their sounding board.

The radiology reports from CT and MRI demonstrated the alarming numbers. Three weeks from the time of the biopsy, the mass increased from 8 cm to 23 cm on the left inferior orbital wall, and the left lateral chest wall increased from 15 cm to 28 cm. Ivan and his family were in complete shock at the diagnosis and how rapidly the soft tissue tumors were growing. Just one month prior, Ivan was still working.

He completed a couple of sessions of palliative radiation to help with pain management. But this was not effective at all. The referral came in as an urgent request from the radiation oncologist to admit him as soon as possible, as his pain was not managed well. Ivan was on extremely low-dose pain medications of oxycodone 5 mg and gabapentin 300 mg, which was not reducing his pain.

This was my first experience with this type of cancer. Undifferentiated Pleomorphic Sarcoma (UPS) is a rare type of cancer that begins mostly in the soft tissues of the body. Soft tissues connect, support, and surround other body structures. Pleomorphic refers to tumors growing in many different shapes and sizes. Symptoms include growing lumps or areas of swelling, neuropathy pain, fever, and weight loss. Ivan had every symptom. UPS accounts for less than 1% of all Cancers diagnosed in adults in the U.S.[18]

I was taken off guard by the appearance of Ivan's back. The tumors were palpable, uniquely shaped, and several inches wide. They had bright red and purple striations on the surface, and the appearance of spider angiomas spread in every direction. The skin was stretched in a rigid fashion.

Every time Ivan tried to turn to his left side, the pain was unbearable, and he would cry out in agony. He lay mostly on his back or right side. The blood vessels were dilated due to the restricted blood flow. I wondered if the tumors might eviscerate through the skin.

Ivan had a temperature of 100.0 Fahrenheit on the first follow-up visit. His oxygen saturation levels were at 88% on room air, and his lung sounds were clear. The family asked questions about the prognosis on the first day, which surprised me. I talked slowly to allow time for interpretation. I located the *Gone From My Sight* book and checked off Ivan's symptoms with them, allowing time for interpretation and questions. Everyone was in shock when I said he most likely had ten days. I didn't mean to upset them, but I knew we had to work quickly so Ivan could have a peaceful transition.

---

[18]   Mayo Clinic, "Undifferentiated Pleomorphic Sarcoma: Symptoms and Causes," https://www.mayoclinic.org/diseases-conditions/undifferentiated-pleomorphic-sarcoma/symptoms-causes/syc-20389554.

The most important item to address was Ivan's pain. He had a difficult time expressing how it felt and giving me descriptors. This is, in my opinion, the number one way to identify neuropathy pain. It tends to present as a very overwhelming and all-encompassing sensation and feeling. Ivan had been taking two of the oxycodone 5 mg tablets every four hours, and it wasn't putting a dent in the pain.

I discussed with the family the medication methadone and how it could help specifically with this type of pain. The term methadone has connotations with the medication used to treat heroin addiction. They were not ready for this prescription. Sometimes, you have to work your way up the ladder. I asked the medical director for a Fentanyl patch, so we started at 25 mcg and quickly titrated to 50 mcg.

I offered a Foley catheter to help so he wouldn't have to use briefs. His response was, 'I'm not an invalid yet!' So, the plan would be to use the urinal or bedside commode.

I asked the family not to do the 20-foot walk to the bathroom as he could desaturate if he took the oxygen off, and the consequences of a fall would be catastrophic. They agreed, but Ivan was strong-willed. I knew we didn't have long to help Ivan, so I asked the family if I could visit every day because the pain was not controlled well.

They would need as much support as possible as they were still accepting the fact that their beloved father and husband was dying of a very rare and terminal cancer. They agreed to the daily visits and said they might cancel on the weekends because it would be a different nurse. I reassured them the on-call nurse would have up-to-date information on Ivan.

Katya did all his personal care and was very devoted to all the details. She did a great job journaling everything, which helped to see how often he was taking oxycodone for breakthrough pain. By four days in, they were more open to learning about methadone and how it helped with neuropathy pain. Ivan described the pain now as burning.

After educating them, they truly wanted Ivan to have less pain as they could see he was getting weaker and closer to being completely bedbound. His initial methadone dose was: methadone 10 mg/ml liquid concentration, one ml two times a day. I explained that we wouldn't see results until day three, most likely, and to keep the Fentanyl patch on for long-acting control until that time. We anticipated possibly titrating every two days as fast as his tumors were growing.

Over the years, I have learned that if the family sees the patient in pain, they are still alive. Barbara Karnes, the Mother Theresa of the hospice movement in America, said it well, "The misconception is that by withholding the narcotic, the person would be alert and interactive. But this is not the case. Either way, the person will become less responsive as their body is shutting down."[19]

Treating the pain can mean that you are accepting of the disease process and what is going to happen eventually. I don't know how else to explain this psychologically, but it is a phenomenon. I clearly saw this with Sasha. I asked her to give him a dose of oxycodone for breakthrough pain during a visit, but she responded crying, "I want him to be more alert and be able to talk with us."

I encouraged her to hold precious those moments he was able to communicate, even if it was just a couple of times per day. I also said, "Your dad is suffering with fast-growing, visible tumors that are truly hurting him, and the pain medication is crucial to bring him comfort."

Working through pain management issues embraces the mental and emotional thought processes of what the family is going through and their beliefs about narcotics. This can be challenging for all people and any culture. It is important to be sensitive and mindful of what the family is experiencing while educating with empathy and truth regarding the disease process. It is our job to advocate for the patient and help the body relax enough to transcend.

Through the following days, Ivan's temperature hovered around 99 to 100 degrees Fahrenheit and was managed with liquid Tylenol. Katya believed in wholesome natural foods and enjoyed making him fruit smoothies and homemade bone broth. Ivan would take a few sips or bites per meal. She also made special teas to help his bowels move. Still, it wasn't quite enough, so she gave the Bisacodyl suppository to help, which was successful.

---

[19] Barbara Karnes, "Does Morphine Hasten Death?" https://bkbooks.com/blogs/something-to-think-about/does-morphine-hasten-death

IN SHOCK

The swelling rapidly spread to the left arm, hands, and shoulder area four plus edema. The day Ivan started the methadone, he rated his pain 7/10. He was taking two (10 mg) oxycodone for breakthrough pain, averaging five times a day, and the Fentanyl was at 50 mcg.

The family called friends and family to update them on Ivan's status. Their pastor came to visit and bring support. They were strong in their faith, and Ivan would acknowledge and point upward. The funeral home decision was made.

Two days after starting the methadone, the pain was down to a better level of 3/10, and he was averaging three doses per day on breakthrough oxycodone. The Fentanyl patch was removed. Methadone slowly took the place of oxycodone tablets for breakthrough pain. His final dosage went to 1 ml of methadone four times a day (40 mg per day). Four days into methadone, Ivan was relaxed and not curled up on his right side for the first time.

I prepared the family for the next step, which would be the Macy catheter. It was difficult for him to swallow, and we could not stop giving him the methadone, or he would have a tremendous pain crisis. They understood the concept of going through withdrawals if narcotics were stopped.

The next day, the on-call nurse came to provide support and placed the Macey catheter for administration of the methadone. She educated the family on administering the medications and flushing the line with water. They declined the Foley catheter and opted for briefs.

When I saw Ivan the next day, he was incredibly peaceful and had slipped into a coma the previous night. His oxygen levels were at 45%. It is amazing when the burden of having to swallow medications is lifted. Another release can happen with the body. The family, including his grandchildren, were showering him with love.

The Aurora led the way with a slow and methodical dance back to Ivan's house at 7 pm. It shimmered in soft shades of aqua and vibrant emerald. Normally, they don't appear until after 11 at night and usually later in the wee hours of the morning. I like to think Ivan let his family know he was dancing with the angels. His body was made whole again after his very brief battle with this rare cancer.

After I pronounced and dressed his body with the help of Katya, multiple family members came and surrounded him with love and tears. The celebration of his legacy lasted throughout the night and into the morning. Then, the family was ready to call the funeral home.

Ivan was on service for eleven days. For these types of rare cancers, where the patient is given a terminal prognosis of weeks to live, it is most beneficial to offer as much support as possible. The family was still in tremendous shock when Ivan started hospice care. Ivan would not have had a peaceful death if he had only been seen two times per week by the nurse case manager, as his pain level was extremely high. It took several days of teaching pain management to the family to achieve a peaceful transition. Ivan was blessed with a family that loved and nurtured him until his final breath.

Hospice Highlights

- Give families time to vent their frustrations and ask questions on day one when it is a new diagnosis.
- Initiate methadone as soon as possible for the "indescribable pain."
- Drill home the concept that whether the person has pain meds or not, they will lose the ability to communicate, and they will become less responsive.
- The patient should receive daily nursing visits until the uncontrolled pain is under control. Consider language barriers and belief systems regarding narcotics in end-of-life care.
- Change visitation plans to meet the needs of the family, particularly in cases with an unexpected diagnosis with rapid decline.

Source

18) Mayo Clinic. "Undifferentiated Pleomorphic Sarcoma: Symptoms and Causes." https://www.mayoclinic.org/diseases-conditions/undifferentiated-pleomorphic-sarcoma/symptoms-causes/syc-20389554.
19) Karnes, Barbara. "Does Morphine Hasten Death?" https://bkbooks.com/blogs/something-to-think-about/does-morphine-hasten-death.

WHITE OUT ON THE SNOW MOON

It was a Snow Moon, and how befitting this title was for the upcoming 15 hours of on-call I endured. I try to make it a habit to go to bed early, around 9 pm, when on call to get a couple of hours of sleep before the falling upward occurrences begin. (Falling upwards is a reference used in hospice nursing, which refers to the common theme that patients experience falls a few weeks before they die.) This is crucial after working an 8-hour day. You need a couple of hours of sleep to keep working through the night. Back in my 20s, this was not a big deal, but at 50, it's a different story.

The first occurrence happened at 1:00 am and then the next at 2:30 am. I had just made it back home to rest and then received the next call at 6:00 am. Of course, the rule of three's applied to the Snow Moon!

The snow had begun falling heavily around 10:00 pm that night, and the inches of accumulation were adding up quickly. It was not just coming down in a gentle, beautiful tapestry, but rather, it was invigorated with side-blowing winds, picking up the snow off the ground, which resulted in low visibility. This is called a ground blizzard. And on the white ground, in the white ground and surrounded by white, is where I spent the next five hours alongside a fellow nurse, EMT personnel, and local townsfolk. But first, let me give you some background on my automobile drama from the previous year.

The year 2021 was challenging, personally and professionally. We were all extremely exhausted from the pandemic. Nursing burnout, being short-staffed, and working in such a politically charged medical crisis was taking its toll on many of us. If that wasn't enough, my Honda Pilot of 17 years died its final death, making it to almost 270,000 miles. This car had served my family well!

So, car shopping I went. I decided on a Toyota Rav 4. It was a 2013 and had 60,000 miles on it. The size was appropriate, and I knew that Toyotas had a good reputation for longevity. But apparently, that was not the case for the 2013 model of this vehicle.

I had just dropped off the nurse I was training at the office and was heading home when I pulled onto the main highway at a very busy intersection. The engine simply just titrated to a quiet rest. I pulled off the road and sat there in the middle of rush hour traffic. I called a tow truck when steam and smoke suddenly started coming out from under the hood.

I wondered how it could be overheating. I knew all the fluids had been topped off. After all, I just bought this car nine days ago! The next thing I knew, smoke was coming inside my car by the armrest console. I did not fully understand what was happening, but I knew this was not normal and got out of the car.

I grabbed my purse and phone and stood in the ditch, away from the highway. I stared in disbelief and shock. People started pulling over quickly and running over to tell me, "It's on fire! Get back, it could explode!"

Someone had already called 911, and within minutes, a fire truck was there dousing water all over my new shiny black car while police officers redirected traffic. I was stunned at the scene taking place. Flames were coming out from the side of the hood and underneath the engine.

I asked the police officer if I could get my computer out of the back seat. He replied, "No, Ma'am, stay back here with me." Fortunately, it was nestled in its bag under nursing supplies, so it didn't get damaged from the copious amounts of water dumped on it to put out the flames in the engine. After that day's events, it put an end to my desire to own a Toyota ever again.

On to the next vehicle. I wasn't sure what to buy, so I used my son's fixer-upper that we had just sunk $2500 into to get it up and running for his first car. He didn't have his license yet, so I had a few months to use it. It was a two-door 2000 Honda Civic with front-wheel drive.

Apparently, my brain was not thinking logically. Front-wheel drive cars in Alaska are not practical at all. After a few near-death experiences, doing 180's on snowy roads in the winter, I was over it. And so was the car, as it also titrated to a quiet rest on my way home from work. At least they all died at the end of the workday!

I test-drove several cars and eventually decided on a Ford Escape with all-wheel drive and fancy buttons for extra traction control. It was reasonably priced, and I even got a rebate for working in the healthcare field. Even though I wasn't a first responder, I told the sales lady I was a *last responder* as a Hospice Nurse. She agreed I should get the rebate. It was smaller, lighter in weight, and had better gas mileage.

Back to the 6:00 am phone call on that Snow Moon. The answering service called, saying the caregiver advised the patient's spouse, Betty, to call 911 because her husband Leo was on the floor and in extreme pain and clutching his left arm. I immediately called Betty and questioned her about what had happened and if she wanted Leo to be comfortable at home or go to the hospital for end-of-life care. She quickly said, "No hospital."

I called EMS back and said we would just need lift support for the patient, and there was no need for lights or sirens. Betty was Leo's power of attorney, and it was confirmed that no transport to the hospital was needed as he was Do Not Resuscitate status.

I asked Betty to give Leo 1 ml of morphine and one tablet of Ativan as his pain was a 10/10 with what most likely was a broken humerus. She said it was swelling quickly, bruised immediately, and was bumpy in appearance. She was instructed to give a dose of meds every 20 minutes until his pain calmed down. I confirmed that his Comfort One form was on the refrigerator in case EMS arrived before we did. We have the caregiver post our state's guidelines so that EMS knows where to find it and can easily see the patient's wishes regarding life-sustaining measures.

Of utmost importance, I refueled with coffee. Then, redressed in snow pants, a coat, a hat, a scarf, and two pairs of gloves with knee-high boots. I grabbed a few snacks and water bottles for the road.

My car was parked outside, not in a garage, as that had been converted to a playroom for my cherubs. In the few hours that I had been home, at least six inches of heavy snow piled up on the car, which required removal. I broomed everything off, got the ice scraper out, and cleared a crunchy layer off the windows.

Off I went, in my downsized, more efficient car. At this point, there was approximately 10-12 inches of snow on the mostly unplowed roads. I stopped midway to get gas and called Betty to say I was en route but very slowly, only driving 35 mph. The main road had only been plowed in one direction, so I drove on the side when no one was coming. Thankfully, they had canceled several schools, so there was not much traffic.

All I could do was pray I would be safe on this journey. I asked for some extra energy as I was running low and to help the patient's pain as he was lying on his bedroom floor waiting for help to arrive. I remember hearing in the back of my mind words from my father, "Plod on, plod on, plod on." It's times like these that you really appreciate the work ethic your parents instilled in you as a child.

Another nurse was also on the way. She knew the family and had been visiting to help with his care. What would normally be a one-hour drive took almost two.

Upon arrival, I saw the ambulance stuck in the road, all lit up like a Christmas tree. The visibility was poor, and the snow was coming down from a side angle. I followed the nurse in front of me, who was paving the way to the patient's house. In the whiteout conditions, we wound up trudging down a path and not a road.

I recall the feeling of slowly sinking. All of a sudden, we were stuck, and I mean, we were stuck beyond comprehension! We were surrounded by deep snow, with a frozen river smack dab in front of us. We got out of our vehicles, and I grabbed two winter hiking poles from the back seat. I gave one to my nursemate, and I took the other. Carrying my nursing bag and a few supplies, we started to trek up the hill.

The trail had a steep grade, and we half walked, half climbed up it as best we could through three feet of heavy, untraveled snow.

We used the trek pole to help keep our balance. As we got to the top of the trail, the EMS guys stood there watching everything. I'm sure they were amused that we were as lost as they were. But at least they got stuck on the top of the ridge.

We all got our bearings, called Betty, and she directed us to her driveway. Finally, we made it to the patient's cabin. Poor Leo had been on the floor now for about 2 ½ hours.

Once inside, Betty showed us to the bedroom. It was obvious that Leo had broken his left arm. It was misaligned, bruised, hot to the touch, and almost double the size of his right upper arm. We medicated him with a dose of morphine before lifting him back into bed since the pain was escalating. We wrapped the left arm in a sling and secured it with duct tape (it's an Alaskan thing).

It took all four of us to get him into the bed, being mindful not to bump into the left arm. I inserted a Foley catheter since turning side to side would be extremely difficult for brief changes now. Leo needed a total of four doses of 1 ml of morphine over the 1.5 hours we were with him to help the pain settle down. He also had an intrathecal pain pump for chronic pain management, which included morphine, baclofen, and clonidine. Finally, he was able to sleep. We sent pictures of the broken humerus to the medical director. He sent a prescription for a Fentanyl patch to the pharmacy to help with long-acting pain control.

The plan was for Leo to pass in his own cabin with his wife and not to be transported to the hospital for treatment. Leo had Parkinson's disease and atherosclerotic heart disease. I spent time talking with Betty about Leo's imminent status now that his oxygen levels were in the 80s and he had broken a major bone. With it not being treated surgically, patients could develop complications of blood clots, fat embolus, or infections and pass away within three to five days. We reviewed the symptoms from *Gone From My Sight,* and Betty chose a funeral home. The case manager brought more meds and the Fentanyl patch on the following day's visit.

At one point, I had to trek back down to my car for more nursing supplies, which took about 30 minutes. Once we had Leo settled, we had to figure out how to get our vehicles unstuck. I called a friend who had a tow truck in town. He refused to help me as he knew his tow truck would get stuck as well. He told me, "You guys are on a trail meant for snowmachines or four-wheelers. Your only hope is to get snow machines to pull you out. Good luck!"

Betty said she would call some friends. The snowmachine saviors were on their way because that's how things work in this town: you help out your neighbors!

They gave us each a ride back to ground zero. They connected a heavy chain and strap to the rear of my car. I was the first to get my adrenaline spiked along with my heart rate. I received some pretty complicated instructions on when to press the gas and how to turn the wheel according to which direction my car would slide.

This was way too much information to process on two hours of sleep. It felt like a horrible geometry problem from high school. Problem-solving with distance, angles, and lines was not my specialty. I have trouble parallel parking and forget it when it comes to backing up situations of this enormity!

I looked in my rearview mirror, trying to process the instructions while simultaneously sticking my head out the window and looking backward through the white fog of smoke and snow. All the while, the snowmachine punched its throttle while chains clanked loud noises, and flumes of smoke circled everywhere.

The snowmachine worked like a muscle car, its raw power pulling a weight four times its own up a steep trail. This went on for at least ten minutes, but I finally made it to the top of the ridge.

Next, it was my nursing partner's turn to be winched up to the top. By this time, a plow truck had pulled the ambulance out, and they were on their way.

After this escapade, I was not satisfied with my choice of a lighter-weight car. This, along with other incidences of me sliding and its poor performance on deeply grooved winter roads, made driving unsafe in snowy situations. We travel to some remote mountainsides, sometimes one-lane roads, and diverse terrain.

The following year, I purchased the Subaru Ascent for its ample room and storage for my big nursing totes and supplies. I am more than happy with its performance in the wintertime. I feel safe and that I'm not going to die in wintertime driving!

Thirteen days later, Leo passed away peacefully with his wife and daughter at his bedside. He survived longer than anyone I've seen thus far, with a major break to the bone that was not treated. He stopped eating five days before passing, and oxygen levels gently titrated down.

We learned a valuable lesson as a team during the "Whiteout on the Snow Moon." Ensure alerts are put into the patient's chart on the computer on admission when the GPS signal ends and written instructions are needed. Entering landmarks is very helpful.

Hospice Highlights

- Keep your car stocked with emergency winter gear, including a small shovel and supplies for patient crises and falls.
- Computer alerts are placed in patient charts when GPS doesn't work and written directions are necessary.
- Have an appropriate Automobile to deal with harsh driving conditions.
- Make sure the POLST form is visible in the patient's home (Physicians Orders for Life-Sustaining Treatment).
- Get sleep when you can for on-call weekends.

GIP: GENERAL INPATIENT LEVEL OF CARE

Ruby was 64 years old with a diagnosis of lung cancer. She had finished the final round of immunotherapy and was glad to be done as it caused severe nausea. She weighed 98 pounds and was a petite five feet tall. Her co-morbidity list included COPD, anxiety, colitis, cachexia, and recent pneumonia.

She recently had an ER visit for an intense bout with colitis and was sent home with several antibiotics, which caused a severe rash. The meds were discontinued due to the rash. Ruby still suffered from frequent loose stools and nausea due to her long history of colitis.

My first meeting with Ruby was 13 days into her being on service. I took over for another nurse case manager as Ruby wanted an older nurse. At the time, I was 49 years old. Sheesh, not even 50, and I was the old one!

I accepted the call for her request. Alongside me was a new nurse practitioner I was training to hospice. We had 100 years between us, so Ruby would be blessed with plenty of "oldness" for our nursing abilities.

Ruby lived in senior housing with many close neighbors. They allowed small pets and smoking, but it had to be done outside in a designated area. Ruby spent most of her time to herself. She was not very social and did not have close friends. Her cat was her best friend, and that was all she needed. The neighbors commented she was a "loner" and would not interact much.

Molly, her daughter, flew up from the lower 48 to be with her mom when it was time for Ruby to go into hospice and needed 24/7 care. She felt obligated as she was her only child. The relationship between mother and daughter was extremely fragile.

We were at the height of the COVID-19 pandemic, which turned our nursing world upside down for many months. I was functioning on autopilot, wondering if I wanted to stay in this profession. With all the media drama surrounding the pandemic and the reality of our work, I got to the point where I couldn't watch the news. It was very difficult to even be in a room with family or friends and talk about the subject because everyone had an opinion and thought they all had the right answers. Yet, none of them understood what it was like to care for a patient dying with COVID.

My experience of caring for those with COVID, along with their terminal disease, was a reality of seeing people die in a state of suspended animation. The patient would often be talking to you one minute and die the next. This was not a normal dying process. The pandemic drama would affect Ruby in her final weeks.

A few days after coming home from the ER, Ruby developed a blood clot in her left arm. Her arm was double in size, cold to the touch, and pale blue with weak pulses. We treated with Aspirin therapy 325 mg by mouth two times a day. We covered her arm with a compression wrap, and in two weeks, it was resolved.

She suffered from nausea, diarrhea, pain, and shortness of breath. She didn't like the taste of the morphine initially, and the struggle with nausea was ongoing, so she took oxycodone, and with three to four breakthroughs per day, she began on the Fentanyl patch at 25 mcg. Even though she was cachectic, it did prove to be helpful for her pain management. Studies have shown that the use of Fentanyl patch compared with oral morphine for long-acting pain management can significantly decrease the occurrence of constipation, nausea and vomiting, and drowsiness.[20]

One week on service, Ruby's anxiety and fear of dying escalated along with her questions. "Was she really dying?" At this point, she

---

[20] PubMed, "Transdermal Fentanyl for Cancer Pain," https://pubmed.ncbi.nlm.nih.gov/29578144.

was ready to revoke hospice and get a second opinion when we contacted the oncologist by phone, and he talked to Ruby. He explained spots were also detected on her liver. This affirmed to her that she should stay in comfort care. I wish I had paid more attention to this little information about liver involvement. Zofran was not helping her nausea, so we started a Scopolamine patch. This proved to help both with nausea and improve Ruby's coarse lung sounds.

On her history and physical, it said she had quit smoking one month prior. That was not the case, as she was smoking when she returned home after the ER visit. She would go outside to smoke, but this would diminish as the weeks progressed with shortness of breath and desaturating escalation. Oxycodone breakthroughs were now averaging five to six per day, so the Fentanyl patch was increased to 50 mcg. Then Ruby had a fall with no injuries.

For Molly to assist her mom through this process, she had to have space at night, so she stayed in a hotel close by. She would come to Ruby's apartment to help set things up in the morning, but they both needed breaks from each other. Molly wanted to get a personal care assistant (PCA) to help with caregiving through grant funding we had access to, but Ruby adamantly refused help from a stranger.

Ruby started to experience sleep disruption when she missed taking a dose of pain meds. She had two more falls, and her blood pressure was low. Then she burnt food while cooking as she got distracted and forgot what she was doing. At this point, I pleaded with Molly to stay with her mom 24/7. She said she would try.

Three weeks into hospice care, Ruby's symptoms were starting to spiral. This was the beginning of her terminal agitation. Molly was with her when oxygen levels dropped to 80%. She was getting more confused, agitated, and extremely irritated. Ruby would not apply the oxygen.

Molly called the on-call nurse to visit. Ruby was so angry that she threatened to call the cops to get Molly removed from her apartment as she was shouting expletives for Molly to leave! By the time the on-call nurse arrived, the local police department was on the scene. Ruby was reaching for intangible things in the air, and her behavior was erratic, but she came back to baseline after oxygen was applied and O2 saturation levels improved. She also started to run a temperature.

The next morning, the nurse practitioner and I visited Ruby and Molly. We talked about safety concerns, as Ruby had to have 24/7 help. Catching the food on fire was extremely unsettling as she lived in a large apartment complex, putting everyone at risk. She was not safe to be alone, not even for five minutes.

Ruby implored, "I need my space, and I want to be alone!" She refused help from her daughter and had yet to give her official power of attorney. We had to make an Adult Protective Service (APS) report for self-neglect as mandatory reporters. Ruby acknowledged what was happening. She was now on daily visits.

Over the next few days, Ruby's behavior calmed down a little, as she knew her brother and sister were flying up to say their goodbyes. Her oxygen levels ranged from mid-70s to 80s, and the oxygen was on and off all day long, not consistent. Ruby allowed Molly to stay with her now while her siblings visited.

After her family left, her vitals deteriorated more, BP 90/70 sats at 78% on four liters of oxygen, and crackles presented in the lungs. She started having severe hallucinations, and then she punched Molly in the face, leaving a noticeable mark. Molly called the on-call nurse, not knowing how to handle her mom's behavior. The nurse gave a nebulizer, and she was willing to take morphine for rescue breathing and to keep the oxygen on. Also, she started on Seroquel that night to help the agitation.

During the visit from us, the old nurses, the next day, we knew the next step was for Ruby to be admitted to the hospital for GIP admission. General inpatient is one of the four levels of care that hospice provides for symptoms that are not manageable in the home setting. Her symptoms were out of control!

There were many reasons why it was not manageable in her home setting, including the fractured relationship between patient and daughter, evidenced by verbal and physical abuse, and the respiratory failure with escalating encephalopathy symptoms. Here is where we circle back to the pandemic drama. The hospital was full and overflowing with patients. We were in a holding pattern for admission.

The on-call nurse was called out again the next night. Ruby had thrown the nebulizer machine against the wall and broken a glass. Molly was in full meltdown as she said she couldn't do this anymore, and she couldn't take her mom's verbal and emotional abuse any longer. The nurse stayed three hours with Ruby and Molly. She gave Ruby meds and tried to keep the oxygen on her.

The morning arrived, and it was our turn to take over. I enlisted my nurse practitioner to be the lucky one to give Ruby the Haldol injection (10 mg) while our medical director was trying to get Ruby a bed assignment. After seven hours of a nursing presence in the home, I called the house supervisor at the hospital, imploring when the bed would be ready. He told me to call back in a few hours and ask again. I about lost my marbles and demanded I be given a bed assignment now. He finally gave me a bed assignment. Non-emergent transport was called, and within 15 minutes, Ruby was at the hospital.

Sometimes, you have to communicate concisely, with authority and professionalism. Ruby needed intravenous and intramuscular meds to manage her symptoms of severe terminal agitation. I know that in big cities where hospices have more employees and are contracted with several pharmacies, they often have access to IV meds in the home setting. This was not the case in our rural location of Alaska.

One would guess Ruby would have passed within a couple of days with oxygen levels in the 70s and all the other symptoms present. That would not be the case. The admitting diagnosis was multiple: acute hypoxic respiratory failure, toxic metabolic encephalopathy, and terminal lung cancer.

Ruby was terrified of dying, and as the days progressed, 12 to be exact, she was on daily nursing visits. We explored the psychosocial and spiritual aspects of who Ruby was. We supported her with chaplain visits, which she received well. We monitored the progress of her symptom management, including Geodon injections, IV Benadryl, IV morphine, IV Ativan, OxyIr tablets, and Fentanyl patch maxed at 200 mcg.

The day after arriving at the hospital, jaundice presented on her skin. Even with all these meds on board, her petite frame managed to get out of bed, and she almost fell in the bathroom. Staff placed a Foley catheter and a bed alarm to alert them if she tried to get up again.

Molly spent most of her time with her mom and took only a few breaks. I thought she was exceptional for staying by her side as she knew her mom was so fearful of dying. Molly said her mom had a lot of regrets and had been bitter about things that happened in her life. She had a faith background as a child, so Molly was happy that the chaplain was visiting.

Three days before Ruby took flight, her sats were at 48% on five liters of oxygen, and her heart rate was at 146. She was sitting up in the hospital bed at a 90-degree angle and said she saw sweet Jesus. She kept saying that phrase over and over again. I asked if we could pray with her, and she nodded. The NP, myself, and Molly prayed that sweet Jesus would take her pain and suffering. Tearfully, we encouraged her that it was okay to release and let go and that she was loved by her daughter, who was by her side. This calmed her down.

The next day, Ruby was nonverbal; however, she was semi-alert and raised her hands upward toward the sky. Mottling had begun. At night, the agitation increased, so the medical director ordered Phenobarbital to help ease her suffering. Ruby passed peacefully the next afternoon in the hospital with Molly by her side, holding her hand. It took *all* forms of medication administration to ease Ruby's terminal agitation, including intravenous, intramuscular, oral, and transdermal meds. The benefits of the general inpatient level of care were critical for Ruby to pass peacefully.

Hospice Highlights

- Advocate with authority.
- Mandatory reporting of abuse/neglect.
- Find reserves when the tank is empty as a nurse.
- General Inpatient Admission is necessary when home management of symptoms cannot be obtained.

Source

20) PubMed. "Transdermal Fentanyl for Cancer Pain." https://pubmed.ncbi.nlm.nih.gov/29578144.

TERMINAL AGITATION

Getting to know Sandy over the course of three months was enlightening as she shared her story. Her diagnosis was hypertensive chronic kidney disease with heart failure. She chose to stop all extensive cardiac medications at the age of 76. Sandy summarized her last few months with clarity and declarative adjectives fitting her spitfire personality.

"Everything happened in the last three years. I started having heart attacks, thirteen to be exact! Every time I had a heart attack, they took me to the cath lab and put one or two stents in my heart, with a total of 21 now. When the doctor put the last stent in, he told me I still had more that needed to be placed, but all the vessels were too little, so they couldn't do it."

Upon receiving that news, she decided to stop cardiac medications and chose care and comfort. How exactly did Sandy come to that decision for care and comfort? It was not attributed to the cardiac doctor as he did not even bring up the idea of hospice. Sandy went to see her physician assistant and told him she wanted a hospice referral.

Who else would do this but a nurse? Sandy had been an LPN for over 50 years. Her final advocation was for herself as the *patient*. Sandy's co-morbidity list was extensive and included congestive heart failure, type 2 diabetes mellitus, atherosclerotic heart disease, atrial fibrillation, coronary angioplasty implant graft, TIA, UTI, cervical cancer, myocardial infarction, obesity, and COPD.

I wanted to get to know this spunky LPN of five decades as she exuded such an unshakeable passion inside of her. Sandy graduated from LPN school in 1965. She told me the story. "Back then, the LPN program was two years long, and you started it your senior year of high school. The starting wage was $1.56 an hour in the hospital setting. I left the hospital setting of ER, OB, and peds and then went to private duty nursing which paid $25.00 per day, $12.00 more per day, which was significant at that time!"

I asked Sandy when she noticed a change in the nursing profession, when the amount of time she could spend with patients became less due to all the regulations. She said that when she moved to Alaska in 2004, she was allowed to do less as an LPN in this state than others. So, she opened up an assisted living facility and ran that for seven years before she quit.

Sandy arrived at the assisted living facility after several weeks in the hospital. She was worn out and glad to be back "home." She had multiple pus-filled blisters on her back and gluteal area. Our medical director suspected it was a pseudomonas infection as the pus was green in color. We healed the blisters with Bactroban ointment and foam pad dressing changes two to three times a week. It took five weeks for them to close over.

Sandy was still enjoying eating even though she had lost over 30 pounds in the past few months. To help her skin condition, we put in a Foley catheter. This helped her skin heal; however, with the history of UTI, these symptoms manifested, so a round of Cipro was started. Three days into Cipro, she was vomiting and experienced severe GI upset, so the antibiotic was discontinued.

Two weeks later, Sandy experienced a raging yeast infection vaginally. The catheter was causing too much discomfort after weeks of flushing it and the infection. We took a break from this intervention, which was no longer helping in any way. A round of oral Diflucan for three days helped to lessen the yeast infection but did not clear it completely. Sandy's main areas of pain were in the chest and legs. Morphine in low dose was administered since that was the best option for cardiac symptoms. Even at a low dose of 0.25 ml (5 mg) a couple of times a day, it caused itching all over her skin. No rashes appeared, just a very annoying itching sensation. To top it off, she was allergic to Benadryl, so we could not use that to treat the itching.

A low dose of Fentanyl patch started at 25 mcg. This worked very well for pain control. We saved the liquid morphine for later if needed. Sandy wore oxygen for comfort, mostly at night, but it became a nuisance, and she didn't care for it.

A common theme from Sandy during our visits was, "How much longer is this gonna take?" I explained to Sandy that since she had stopped all her cardiac meds, it would most likely be weeks to a few months' prognosis. I also shared that nutrition keeps one alive and that when all nutritional intake stops, it is usually a 7 to 10-day process before breathing and the heart stops. But Sandy still enjoyed eating, so I encouraged her to eat or drink whatever she liked. Still, it was her choice to keep doing so, which was keeping her body alive. She understood.

We also talked about the spiritual and emotional elements of the dying process and how they were just as significant as the physical symptoms she was experiencing. Sandy was strong in her faith and had peace in this area of her life. However, Sandy was a type A personality. She knew how to be the boss and be in charge. She was telling her physical body she was still in charge! Even though each week she would claim she "was ready to go," she still wasn't ready to surrender on the emotional and spiritual levels. Though her body was crying out to be released, her soul would not surrender.

I cannot emphasize enough how important it is for hospice nurses to develop trust with our patients as we care for them. Trust is established by being open and honest with communication, being authentic with how you deliver care, and showing empathy and kindness to your patient. Having knowledge of pain and symptom management and explaining this to your patient is critical. Once trust is established, the ability to have hard conversations about the dying process can begin on every level. Being effective in our hospice nursing practice involves more than taking vital signs and asking our patients about their levels of pain and when their last bowel movement was.

The personal story that unfolds is amazing and beautiful. One can compare this exquisiteness to seeing new life enter this world. A baby has hope for a future, learning how to love, chase after dreams, experience joy, make mistakes and learn from them. At the end of our human existence, all of these elements that we have developed can be presented in a beautiful story. It doesn't negate the fact there may be suffering, pain, and sadness, but who we are and how we have grown will shine through.

This brilliant display may be a positive or negative experience. The opportunity for family and friends to engage in this final tapestry of life is a beautiful gift to be a part of. Seeing your patients more than once weekly is vital to cultivating this relationship with them.

One reason why I saw Sandy three times a week from the beginning was because her daughter, Sarah, was running the ALF. It was very hard for Sarah to do all the personal care for her mom as she was terminal. It took an emotional toll on Sarah. Offering more support with symptom management is not the only reason for the nurse case manager to increase visit frequency. We can't underestimate how family members cope as the primary caregiver. Sarah was caregiving for six other clients living in the home.

Sandy's love of food gave us many delightful stories to share. She enjoyed eating three meals a day plus snacks, especially biscuits and bread. She told me about the different types of jams and jellies she preferred, and we compared notes on the best recipes.

A gold mine of lingonberries (low bush cranberries) was not too far from where she lived. These berries are my favorite and very easy to pick; just a lot of crawling on the ground. It was mid-September, and the first frost had just occurred. The berries were beckoning to be picked.

At the end of the day, I donned my rain pants and picked up Daisy, our Goldendoodle, and off to lingonberry land we went. I picked a gallon so I would have enough to make a few batches of jam on the weekend. Picking berries with no one around you but your canine to keep you company and protect you is another wonderful form of nature therapy. This helped me to decompress from all the emotions and challenges I experienced throughout the week. Sandy was thrilled when I brought her a few jars of jam the next week. She enjoyed the tangy, tart, sweet treat with her morning biscuits.

Sandy was also very independent and often said things like, "I gotta make it to see my church get into their new building" or "I wanna get up in that chair again." I explained that it had been over two months in the hospital bed, and her body was severely deconditioned. We would have to use a Hoyer lift to get her to the chair, and there was no room in the bedroom to use one. She listened but then would ask me later if we could try again. Repeating answers to her questions and then diverting to another topic was often key in my communication with Sandy.

As we approached almost 2 1/2 months into service, Sandy's pain increased, and titrations of Fentanyl patch reached 100 mcg. Sarah noticed a change in her behavior, with being more verbally feisty than normal and shaking the bedrails while trying to get out of bed. Sarah believed this was a reaction to the increase in Fentanyl.

I gently explained to Sarah this could be the beginning of terminal agitation, but we could decrease the Fentanyl since she felt strongly that this was the cause. I needed Sarah to understand exactly what was transpiring so we could move forward with more effective medication management once she realized it was TA. I decreased the Fentanyl back to 50 mcg.

Three days later, Sarah called in the morning to tell me that the behaviors were more intense and that I needed to come over now rather than later in the day to assess them. It was very clear her original behaviors had nothing to do with a reaction to increasing the Fentanyl. We were now in full-blown TA symptoms. Not only had she been shaking the bed rails, but she managed to get her legs over the side and half fell out onto the floor. Per the doctor's orders, the Fentanyl was increased back to 100 mcg, and Lorazepam 0.25 ml 4 x day was prescribed. We discontinued the Xanax tabs as her ability to swallow pills was diminishing.

The factors that led up to Sandy's last few weeks were multifactorial. Her personality was one of great perseverance through the challenging times of her life. She had been married several times and lived in many different states. She saw the face of nursing change over five decades. Through it all, her faith was deep and sincere. This was her foundation.

Sandy was seen daily for her last 18 days to help with symptom management and support Sarah. Fentanyl titrated up to 200 mcg. The "heaviness of just being in bed" were some of the words she used to describe what she was feeling. An interesting symptom these last few weeks was Sandy's left leg, which developed edema overnight from one plus to four plus, pitting edema, groin to feet. Her pulses were very weak, and her skin temperature was cold. It appeared to be a blood clot, but then it tapered down to two plus edema, and it was not painful for us to move her leg while repositioning in bed.

Sandy was unable to talk at this point, but she would open her eyes slightly as we worked with her and re-positioned her. We decided to put the Foley catheter back in as we knew she only had a few days left, as evidenced by decreasing oxygen saturation levels. We believed this might help her relax even more. Her chaplain from church came one more time. A Kennedy's ulcer appeared on her coccyx the day before she took flight. Sarah was relieved to know Sandy's journey was almost over. She just wanted her mom to be free and be in Heaven.

Sandy experienced Terminal Agitation symptoms for a total of 22 days before she died. Doubling the Fentanyl patch helped, as well as low-dose liquid Ativan every six hours and as-needed morphine before performing bed care. We used several non-pharmacological modalities, such as low lighting in the room, therapeutic touch and gentle massage, and switching the TV channels from news to more peaceful ones. Sandy liked to listen to the news all day, but when the TA symptoms started, I changed the channel!

It took 86 days for her journey to be complete once she stopped all of her cardiac medications. Supporting Sandy and her daughter Sarah with daily visits during those final weeks was critical to ensure effective symptom management, encourage spiritual support, and release Sandy to take flight. I remember saying goodbye to Sandy on a Monday visit and recalled what she had told me early on: *"I know what's waiting for me; it's in His hands, so we gotta let him do His work."* She passed peacefully that night.

Hospice Highlights

- Assessing the ability and available personal resources of caregivers.
- Allow patients and caregivers to be part of the decisions regarding medications.
- Non-medical comfort care, TV channel switch, and low-lighting for terminal agitation.
- Terminal agitation duration can vary from days to several weeks.

SEISMIC 7.1

It was Friday, November 30, 2018. We made it to the end of the workweek in anticipation of a relaxing weekend, *except* I had on-call that night. So, my rest and relaxation would not start until 8 am Saturday.

The nursing staff gathered in the hallway, getting ready to enter our little office and start our stand-up report from the previous night. At 8:29 am, we felt powerful and violent shaking. Five seconds in, one of the supervisors shouted at the top of her lungs, "EARTHQUAKE!"

The first one to exit our lower-level office was a physical therapist. They ran to the door and out of the building like a cheetah. As things were flying off the shelves and coming down around me, I followed her lead. There was no way I was staying on the lowest level of this two-story antiquated building, trying to find something to duck and cover from the ambush of falling debris. I did not want to be buried alive!

It was the weirdest sensation, running as fast as you could while the earth was moving in giant waves underneath your feet. Trying to stay vertical while balancing was almost impossible. Not one person stayed inside the building, standing in a doorway or under a desk.

Around thirty seconds later, the shaking stopped. Dozens of our staff stood outside the building in shock at what had just transpired. Different parts of the valley felt it longer than we did. According to the USGS, it lasted under one minute.

Here in Alaska, we are used to earthquakes as there are four major fault systems that run through the state. However, this quake rattled everyone to the core! After experiencing this seismic activity, I'm sure many people updated their emergency preparedness plans.

My first thought was that my precious niece, Maddy, had just arrived from South Carolina. She was 13 at the time and was home alone in my house. I quickly called and told her to get out of the house with the dog and stay there until I came home.

As I jumped into my car, my boss asked if I was okay. I said, "Yes, but I needed to scoop up my children and niece and deliver them to my mom's house before I could do any work." Everyone was verifying their family members were safe. Then, we proceeded to go through the call list of patients to check in on everyone and initiate our emergency protocol.

My sister Beth was with my mom when it hit. What a blessing she was there to help. She recounts crawling on the floor, heading in the direction of where my mom was as things were crashing down around her. She yelled at her from the opposite end of the house to stay in the laundry room and not move. They had more damage due to the epicenter only being 10 miles from their house.

Long-time residents of Alaska said this was the strongest earthquake Alaska had experienced since 1964. The 1964 quake registered as the most powerful in North America at 9.2 on the Richter scale. That one continued for four minutes and 38 seconds. There was tremendous devastation to Anchorage, and coastal towns were destroyed by the Tsunami and the loss of over 100 lives.[21]

I arrived at my home, and Maddy was quite the trooper standing outside with our Schnauzer, Rupert. Rupert, on the other hand, was a hot mess. I medicated him quickly with Trazodone. Maddy was calm on the phone with her mom, who was at Granny's house nine miles away.

We went inside to inspect the damage. We couldn't smell any gas leaks and didn't have any major items displaced; just some plants and dishes were damaged, and there was a mirror on the floor. We gathered some emergency preparedness bags, extra clothes, and Rupert's anxiety meds, and off we went to Granny's.

---

[21] The New York Times, "Anchorage, Alaska Earthquake," https://www.nytimes.com/2018/12/01/us/anchorage-alaska-earthquake.html.

SEISMIC 7.1

I wanted the teens safe with Aunty and Granny so I could work through the night without worrying about them in the house alone. What was yet to come was more traumatizing than the initial earthquake, the aftershocks. Over 80 aftershocks of various magnitudes were recorded throughout the day, with at least three having magnitudes greater than 5.0. By December 3rd, 170 aftershocks with a magnitude over 3.0 had been noted. It was exhausting to run outside after these aftershocks. By the second day, I would just wait, hold still, and assess.

My daughter, Bella, left school early as she had just gotten her driver's license. The teachers tried to stop her from leaving, but she replied in a determined fashion, "You know no schoolwork will be done today. I have the right to leave, and I'm going to be with my family." A friend delivered Simon, my son, to Granny's house.

Upon entering my mom's home, it was just unbelievable the damage that occurred with, furniture and bookshelves toppled over, grandfather clock on the ground, paintings, and shattered glass all over the floor. Structurally, the house was sound and had no leaks. Thankfully, Beth was in charge of ordering everyone into cleanup mode. But first, it took them a few hours to process and call other family members to let them know we were all safe.

Off I went back to work. There was no need for extra coffee that day as we all had ample adrenaline running through our systems. Every case manager was responsible for calling their patients to check their status. I started by calling my patients to check in with those I could reach by phone. I crossed the names that my CNA was able to get ahold of off my list. I made sure those who had oxygen had electricity. Thankfully, those with no electricity and were on continuous oxygen had backup generators. A few patients had to be relocated for respite care in our contracted facility because they had no electricity.

Some patients were unreachable by phone, so we checked on them in person. We took meals, water, and heaters for those who needed this assistance. One of the nurses on our team offered to do the first death call that came in around 1 pm since she was close by to my patient. I knew the rule of threes would be in play on this epic day. My first visit was in the late afternoon for death call number two. The family was prepared and had good support from children who lived close by.

It was impossible to get decent sleep that night with the ongoing aftershocks. I woke up exhausted. My next death call came in around 7:30 am. This patient lived closer to the epicenter. The roads I needed were travelable. I avoided the main connecting road to the two ends of town as it was completely impassible.

When I arrived, the son needed to process it, so he told me the story of what happened. He said, "When the shaking started, I was in another room. I ran quickly to my mom's room because the T.V. was on the wall directly above her head. I knew it was not hung securely. I just covered my mom with my whole body, and the T.V. came crashing down on my back and broke into pieces. Mom was already in a coma, and she didn't flinch." She passed peacefully that morning. He was so thankful she wasn't hurt, and he only acquired a few cuts and scratches on his back from the incident.

One nurse who lived in Anchorage at the time recalled, "I was at work when it happened and went immediately back home to my husband and baby. Just a few minutes after the quake, the tsunami warnings started coming in, telling people in our area to seek higher elevations. We looked out our living room window, and we were completely gridlocked in.

Cars were lined up on all the streets around our house, sitting at a standstill. We couldn't have left even if we wanted to unless we went on foot. I packed a couple of emergency bags, and we hunkered down at home all day. Meanwhile, I fielded calls from our patients and helped everyone activate their emergency plans."

It was a miracle that there were no fatalities from this earthquake. 117 were reported to have minor injuries, some with broken bones, but there were no deaths reported. When you looked at the devastation that occurred on several roads and the inside of buildings, it was astonishing to comprehend. The damage to buildings and roadways through the valley and Anchorage was estimated to be over $76 million.[22] A federal disaster was declared shortly after the earthquake.

---

[22] Anchorage Daily News, "The Tally of Anchorage Buildings Significantly Damaged by the Quake Surpasses 750 and Counting," https://www.adn.com/alaska-news/anchorage/2018/12/30/the-tally-of-anchorage-buildings-significantly-damaged-by-the-quake-surpasses-750-and-counting/

SEISMIC 7.1

> **HOSPICE HIGHLIGHTS**
>
> - Have emergency supplies ready in your vehicle and at your residence for various disasters.
> - Know your company's policy for the emergency protocol and triage for your patients.

Source

21) The New York Times, "Anchorage, Alaska Earthquake," https://www.nytimes.com/2018/12/01/us/anchorage-alaska-earthquake.html.
22) Anchorage Daily News."The Tally of Anchorage Buildings Significantly Damaged by the Quake Surpasses 750 and Counting." https://www.adn.com/alaska-news/anchorage/2018/12/30/the-tally-of-anchorage-buildings-significantly-damaged-by-the-quake-surpasses-750-and-counting/.

THE LOVE OF A SISTER

My first visit with Mae was at her kitchen table accompanied by her husband Frank. Mae was quiet and not one for many words. She had just awoken and was dressed in her housecoat and slippers, her hair disheveled. Her husband did most of the talking as he was in control of all of her care. Mae would answer my questions, but they were very brief. My first thought was that this was her personality, that she was more introverted and shy.

Mae's pain was mostly in her right lung area and back. She scored it a 5/10. Her oxygen levels measured 88% on room air, so I set up the oxygen to three liters, and she climbed to the mid-90s. Mae was agreeable to try this for comfort measures and also to begin liquid morphine at a small dose of 0.25 ml. I asked Frank to record every time she took the medication so I would have a good picture for my next visit. He agreed to do so.

Mae's diagnosis was breast cancer with metastasis to the lung and bones. She was diagnosed with breast cancer ten years prior and underwent a mastectomy with radiation following. She was in full remission until this past year, when the cancer spread to her lungs and bones. Co-morbidities included malignant pleural effusion, hypertensive heart disease with heart failure, previous alcohol use, anxiety, and bipolar disorder. It is important to become mindful and pay attention to all co-morbidities listed in the patient's history. These can, at times, take a dominant lead in how things develop with your patient as time moves forward.

I noticed Frank's speech was like someone recovering from a stroke. I didn't know what to make of it, but most of his words were clear, and he was at least functional in the house. He showed me around the house so I could see how far Mae had to walk from her bedroom to the bathroom and to locate the best place for the oxygen concentrator.

The POLST (non-resuscitation) form had not been signed yet, so this would be a topic for upcoming visits. Sometimes, you must only tackle a few items per visit. Frank said he wanted Mae to make that decision, but she was not ready. A few days later, after discussing what would happen if Mae fell and Frank called 911 for intervention to go to the hospital, Mae was agreeable to signing the POSLT.

The following week, Mae said the morphine was too strong and made her sleepy and nauseous. So, the medical director wrote for hydrocodone. She tolerated this better with Ibuprofen three times a day at mealtime for the bone pain she was experiencing.

Frank wanted a lockbox for the narcotics for safety. He was concerned Mae might get confused and take too much, even though he was the one giving the medication. I filled the med box weekly.

Mae had questions about whether she should be seeing her psychiatrist in Anchorage. I explained now that she was in hospice care, the medical director could order the anxiety meds. Traveling two-plus hours for that visit would be very challenging in her current condition with her pain and need for continuous oxygen. She allowed me to fill her med box with her anxiety medications. She was worried about running out. I assured her I would not let that happen.

After Mae had been on service for five weeks, she called her sister Daphne for help. She had kept things quiet for long enough and knew she could no longer hide what was happening in her home. Upon my arrival, Daphne was present, and she had a brochure that she presented to Frank for AA (Alcoholics Anonymous) and told him that he needed to get a sponsor. Frank was crying, very emotional, and apologizing.

He had been drinking more, hence the altered speech I had observed weeks prior! I never suspected this because any time I sat next to him at the table for a visit, I never smelled alcohol on his breath. Our social worker came with me to the next visit. Frank refused to get a sponsor and said he was okay. He wasn't.

I was on call that weekend when I received a call from Daphne. She said Frank was found at the local grocery store early in the morning. He had fallen, hit his head, and was unconscious and unresponsive. He underwent brain surgery and was on a ventilator for life support. They couldn't take him off sedation due to the withdrawal symptoms from alcohol he experienced. He was completely out of the picture now.

To my surprise, Mae was relieved! She told the social worker on the next visit with her that he was emotionally and verbally abusive towards her, and this had been going on for many years. When the hospital called asking Mae to make decisions for Frank, she told them she would not, and they needed to call his family. With Mae's permission, we spoke to the nurse practitioner involved in Frank's care on speaker phone together. I explained that Mae was in hospice, and she had enough dealing with her own diagnosis. Mae made it very clear she wanted nothing more to do with her abusive husband.

Daphne came to the nursing visit the next day, and we came up with a plan for the following weeks until we could figure out an assisted living facility placement. Daphne became Mae's Power of Attorney for healthcare. My nursing visits increased to three times a week, and the social worker visited on the two days a week I did not come.

It was interesting to see Mae's pain symptoms improve greatly once Frank was out of the home. She now rated it at a 1/10. Her countenance was lighter, and she was starting to smile. She even showed me some of the oil paintings she had done throughout the years. She was so proud of her artwork.

Mae was living by herself with agency help starting in a few weeks. So, we set things up to be as safe as possible with a bedside commode in her bedroom, an oxygen concentrator for nighttime use, and a lifeline necklace to help assist her if she fell. For safety, I set the meds up in her med planner for only two days at a time, and the rest were in the lockbox.

A few days later, Mae started to experience nausea and fever. We tried the Scopolamine patch, which had to be removed due to extrapyramidal side effects. A hospital bed and more equipment were ordered. The nausea eventually subsided.

Due to ongoing short-staffing issues with caregiver agencies during the Pandemic, there was no help available from several agencies. We were in a predicament as Daphne lived in two different states managing her business. Mae did not want to live with any other family members. Her anxiety increased now with growing confusion and resistance to wearing the oxygen.

Christmas was approaching as we reached the pinnacle of the shortest days of sunlight. This affects one's symptoms of seasonal affective disorder and bipolar symptoms. Depression can manifest in many ways.

Daphne called to tell me Mae was hearing three voices in her head telling her to kill herself. I notified the medical director of the situation and quickly went over. He informed me this had happened back in the springtime, and she had to be hospitalized to stabilize her psychiatric medications. When daylight hours rapidly increase in springtime, mental conditions can often be exacerbated, manifested by anxiety, mania, and other symptoms specific to the psychiatric condition.

Daphne signed the revocation form from hospice and took her directly to the ER for evaluation. I gave the ER Doctor a full report and all the necessary paperwork of POA, medication list, history and physical, Certificate of Terminal Illness (CTI), and POLST. She was admitted and stayed in the hospital for three days. In the meantime, Daphne had time to keep looking for an assisted living facility placement.

December can be a challenging month for Alaskans who struggle with Seasonal Affective Disorder and other psychiatric conditions due to the lack of sunlight experienced during this month. By December 21st, South Central Alaska receives 5 hours and 36 minutes of daylight, with sunrise at 10:08 am and sunset at 3:44 pm. The lack of sunlight means less serotonin, and this can affect one's mood.

After December 21st, we start increasing slowly with more seconds, then minutes, then hours, to a culmination on June 21st of 19 hours and 28 minutes of light. The sun rises at 4:16 am and sets at 11:44 pm. I guess you could say that living in Alaska is like living in a bipolar state. It is a land of extremes with longer dark winters and excessive light during the short summers.

We tend to play hard in the summertime with many pursuits. As the winter months progress, it becomes easier to stay indoors unless you are inclined to outdoor activities. For the elderly, walking in the snow and ice is very challenging, especially with mobility and safety. The feeling of isolation increases since it is difficult to maneuver outside. I believe the extreme darkness exacerbated Mae's bipolar condition.

I have never seen a family member take charge with such decisive action, compassion, love, and hard work in my entire Hospice career. The actions that Daphne demonstrated were beyond amazing. When she knew it was impossible to hire help to keep Mae in her own home, she started visiting all the ALFs in the area. There were not many openings. She found a place that had a room on the independent side, which meant she would still have to find hired help 24/7 as Mae was declining.

This seemed impossible as we couldn't even get help from established agencies. It would have to be a private hire. At the same time, Daphne prepared Mae's residence for sale to pay for the ALF costs and private hire Certified Nursing Assistants. The love for her sister that Daphne had for Mae will forever be imprinted in my heart.

How did she manage to do this? She offered double the wages. Daphne was quite the businesswoman and knew how to get the job done! Later, one of these CNAs came to work for our agency as she developed a passion for end-of-life care. Everything happens for a reason. Sometimes, we see the immediate fruit, and other times, it is in the future.

Mae was happy to be living in a new place with distant memories of Frank. Daphne bought her a few new items to spruce up the place and make her feel more comfortable. Mae was only in her apartment for a little over three weeks when her symptoms increased with shortness of breath, anxiety, and more bone pain.

Norco was increased to 10 mg four times a day, and she needed the oxygen continuously to maintain low 90s saturation levels. The shortness of breath escalated quickly, and it was severe. I explained to Mae her body was starting the final process of decline. She had a hard time accepting this, as Frank made so many decisions for her and controlled her for so long.

She asked me if this really was happening. I explained that from everything I understood and knew, yes, it was her time. She wanted to be sure and see if anything else could be done. So, she revoked hospice care and went to the ER. Our medical director was there and did a chest x-ray, which revealed pleural effusion and severe tumor progression in both lungs. He drained 150 cc of fluid off the lungs, but no permanent drain was placed.

The M.D. thoroughly explained her disease progression to both Mae and Daphne and answered all their questions. They understood and were at peace now. The order to readmit to hospice was sent, and Mae came back on service.

Mae was mobile those last few days but became weak. I placed a Foley catheter as she was unable to void her last 18 hours, causing her to become restless. Liquid morphine and liquid Ativan were a good combination the last couple of days for shortness of breath and pain as she slipped into a deep sleep. Daphne was faithful until the very end, by her sister's side. Oh, the love of a sister! There is nothing that can compare.

HOSPICE HIGHLIGHTS

- Be mindful of all the Co-morbidities of your patient and understand their background.
- There is a purpose for revocation and re-admission to Hospice.
- Support the POA in the change of living situation with the patient. Engage the entire team.
- When appropriate, ask for private time with the patient to assess if the patient may be in an abusive relationship with the caregiver.

THE GOOD SAMARITAN

At 11 am on Wednesday, they patiently waited in the ICU discharge room for oxygen to be delivered so Waylen could be transported home safely. Bea had known Waylen since she was a baby, and he was her dad's best friend. She even referred to him as Uncle Waylen.

So much had transpired over the past several weeks, and Bea needed time to process it. However, hospital discharges can be tedious, and there was no time to think about the journey that lay ahead of her. By 3 pm, the equipment provider had not shown up with the oxygen set up. Bea talked with the nurse again only to find out the order had *just* been sent to the equipment company, even though they signed discharge paperwork at 11 am.

Authorizations from insurance companies can take time to process, and she knew that insurance companies closed at 5 pm. So, Bea took matters into her own hands and got on the phone with Medicaid to pay for it herself until Medicaid could authorize this expense.

How did Bea know to do this? The discharge planner certainly didn't explain it. Because she worked in medical billing, she understood the delays that could occur with Medicaid. By 5 pm, Waylen was set up with a portable oxygen tank for transport home and left the hospital for the last time.

Waylen was a tough, reclusive Alaskan man used to living on his own. He lived in a remote area, in a small cabin far from town. He never married or had children. He worked remotely in several parts of the state doing construction-type work. He also worked on the iconic tram building project at Girdwood Ski Resort. His exposure to many harsh chemicals over the years explained most of his diagnosis. Waylen was thankful Bea had taken him into her home for however long he needed. His gratitude was quiet and soft-spoken. The bond between these two had been decades in the making.

Upon arrival at Bea's home, the equipment company set Waylen up with the oxygen concentrator for in-home use. The next morning, he was admitted to hospice. The admitting diagnosis was acute respiratory failure with hypoxia. His comorbidity list was quite extensive, which included acute kidney failure, pulmonary hypertension, right heart failure, atrial fibrillation, emphysema, and chronic pain.

I met Waylen the day after admission, and I was quite happy to see Bea again! This was not the first time Bea was a caretaker for a family member.

Waylen, a stout and tall man, sat on the couch eating his breakfast with oxygen on at three liters. He would easily get short of breath with any exertion of energy, getting up from the chair, walking, anything. We talked about using morphine with a low starting dose of 0.25 ml before getting up and moving for air hunger. This did provide some relief. But we had a long way to go for Waylan to trust using morphine as a helping agent, as Waylen had stern beliefs about our medications in the USA and where they originated from—the Far East.

At the end of my first visit, Bea and I talked outside. She asked how long I thought he had. I explained the severity of his shortness of breath and the fact that he had become oxygen-dependent within just a few days' time. It could be a six-week or less prognosis. My gut was telling me less, like 2 to 3 weeks, and I should have emphasized that more.

Within three days, Waylen had climbed to 10 liters of oxygen for the extreme air hunger and used morphine and liquid Ativan together to help with symptom management. Bea felt that having the oxygen on that high of a level was like a false sense of security for Waylen. She said it was shocking to see how rapidly his breathing deteriorated. Within days, he went from eating and walking to becoming bedbound.

Four days after admission, on a Sunday, Bea called the on-call nurse for a visit as his air hunger symptoms increased. Morphine and liquid Ativan were increased. The need for a power of attorney for healthcare was of great importance as his decline accelerated. Waylen's brother, Lance, who lived out of state, and Bea would share POA.

Waylen was ready for the hospital bed, and the order was placed for Monday morning (he strongly refused this on admission.) I notified the medical director of the need for a Fentanyl patch as well. Waylen was placed on daily nursing visits to help manage the increasing respiratory symptoms and anxiety.

Bea had found a will in a packet of paperwork from Waylen's house. It indicated that Waylen was married and had children. It even had names listed. Her heart about stopped, and she phoned her dad immediately. Her father verified that it was not accurate.

Upon further inspection, Bea found it was a sample pre-filled page that Waylen had started to write out many years ago. It had information about a sample family on the pre-filled page. After she collected herself, Bea downloaded information and prepped the official POA and last will and testament paperwork. The notary came to the house for the signing the next day.

Waylen knew he was declining rapidly. He gave permission for Bea to look through his phone for contacts so she could let his friends know what was happening. The name Jake came up several times on his recent call list. She called him and found out that he was a former co-worker and friend. Waylen originally wanted to sell his Pontoon boat to Jake but then decided to give his boat to him.

They used to fish together and had great memories on his boat. They planned to spread his ashes from a special location in the pontoon boat. It was very important for Waylen to make these arrangements before his passing and bring closure to the things dear to his heart.

The hospital bed arrived, and Waylen agreed to try it to help elevate his head and ease his breathing. We waited to apply the Fentanyl patch until the next night after Waylen's estranged brother of 10 years, Lance, arrived for a visit. He wanted to be as alert as possible.

His brother stayed for four days. He had questions about if Waylan was really dying or if he would get better. It felt awkward for Bea to see the interaction between the two brothers, knowing he had not been a part of his life for so many years. Bea continued to extend her hospitality as Lance stayed in her home for those four days.

It was a bustling household with her two children under five years of age, caring for her dying adopted uncle and welcoming his estranged brother into her home. She managed to fit in work hours through the wee hours of the morning with her medical billing job. Normally, she would stay up until 2 am working online, but now, she was juggling tending to Waylen's needs with her work routine. Her best friend came over several times to help out with the kids when needed, and her faithful husband worked with schedules to keep moving forward.

Waylen had a fall out of the bed a few days after it arrived; he thought he was strong enough to maneuver himself. After this, Bea stayed in the room with him at night and slept on a mattress on the floor next to him. She could keep a close eye on him and administer the liquid meds more easily.

The Fentanyl patch was doubled by day three to 100 mcg as the amount of liquid morphine he was taking warranted the increase. Waylen broke out in a mild rash on the abdomen and chest area, which we treated with Benadryl cream. Sometimes narcotics can cause mild rash and are easily treatable with creams or Benadryl.

He was beginning the visioning process and seeing people in the hallway waiting for him. All the while, his oxygen saturation levels maintained 97% on 10 liters of oxygen while he experienced 25-second periods of apnea. When the chaplain visited that day, he asked, "How can I pray for you?" Waylen replied, "That the pain would stop."

The next day, the restlessness increased, and the Ativan and morphine weren't enough, so Haldol liquid was added. I like to call this the *HAM Cocktail,* as it is quite effective when terminal agitation sets in. All these medications enhanced one another and were effective when given in the prescribed dosages.

After Lance left, we knew it would be easier to place the Foley catheter. Lance struggled to accept that Waylen was in the dying process, and giving Waylen a catheter was more evidence his body was shutting down. The catheter would make his overall care easier as it was getting too difficult to apply the briefs, and needing to lower the head of the bed was not good for his breathing. After it was placed,

Waylen settled into a deeper sleep, and amazingly, saturation levels were maintained in the high 90s.

The next day, it was too difficult for Waylen to swallow the meds. Even with the slow absorption by mouth, it gave him coughing fits, so the on-call nurse placed the Macey catheter, which worked very well. It was good timing for what transpired the next morning.

The next morning, new symptoms displayed in a dramatic fashion. Bea was absolutely stunned, to say the least! She was not expecting projectile vomiting that landed all over her body and several feet across from her to the bedroom wall. She fumbled for the Yonkers suction machine to clear his throat, but the mess was already everywhere. She phoned the answering service, and the on-call nurse, Sarah, responded.

She called me as she was new to hospice and still learning the dynamics of crisis symptom management. I encouraged her on the basics. The head of the bed must stay at a 60-degree angle, and when she arrived to give the liquid meds (HAM cocktail) after placing the Macey catheter. The Scopolamine patch was already in place behind his ear for secretions. I called the pharmacy and ordered Phenergan suppositories to help settle his GI tract. (Suppositories can be administered right next to the Macey catheter.)

I arrived about an hour after Sarah. The liquid meds were administered every 15 minutes for a 2-hour period. Waylen settled into a quiet rest, with his respirations not so labored. His oxygen saturation levels were in the 70s.

Bea's sister came over, and they talked with Waylen's mom on the phone to update her. They thought it would be special for her to have a print of his hand, so they painted his hand blue and made a print on canvas for his mom to have. They sat next to Waylen and told him they loved him and that it was okay to let go now. Waylen took his last breath with his two adopted nieces by his side. He was finally at peace, and his chronic pain was gone.

After the funeral home received Waylen into their care, Bea felt emotionally and physically over it. She went to Hydrate Alaska for some vitamin B therapy. They put her in a private room, and the rejuvenation therapy was well received. The nurse who administered the IV bag was so gracious to her and said, "This one is on me today after everything you've been through." The tears poured even more as she released so many emotions.

A few weeks after Waylen had passed, I spent some time with Bea. She opened up about everything that transpired before Waylen came home with her for his last few weeks of life. It was heartwarming to see her process her anger, frustration, sadness, and decisiveness so intimately as she talked about the journey that led up to the hospice admission.

Two months prior, Waylen had made several trips to the emergency room for shortness of breath. They gave him the diagnosis of emphysema, tuned him up with oxygen and nebulizer treatments, and sent him home with only inhalers and no permanent oxygen setup. After an appointment with the cardiac doctor, he was so short of breath that he called Bea to drive him home. He was told that he needed to see the pulmonologist, and they were supposed to call him for an appointment.

A few days later, Bea checked in on Waylen. Again, he was so short of breath, with panic in his voice, saying, "I can't breathe! I can't breathe!" She called 911 to get him to the hospital. The ER doctor assured him that they would get his breathing under control but still wanted to send him back home. Then, something happened, and they decided to run more tests.

At the time, Bea had gone to the store and bought him some clothes as he was wearing very worn-out clothing. When she returned to the ER, the doctor said, "Waylen is staying, and we are admitting him to the ICU." The pulmonologist and cardiologist explained that he had a hole in his heart that never fused together. He had a long laundry list of problems, and they wanted to send him to Seattle for further testing and treatment. Waylen said no, as he'd had enough. The doctors then offered hospice referral for comfort measures.

Bea needed to process the feelings of anger towards the medical community, for lack of better words, for not giving serious thought to a man in his 60s with a homely appearance entering the ER. Why did they send him home in the state he was in without admitting him for a diagnostic workup after the first ER visit? Why did the Cardiologist send him home with low oxygenation levels and not send him to be admitted to the hospital?

These are questions Bea will never get answered. Expressing emotions and being raw with your feelings during the grieving process is the first step to letting go of frustration and anger. Our natural emotions are meant to be felt and experienced. Being able to forgive can take time.

Hospice Highlights

- Use a high-flow oxygen concentrator for Respiratory failure diagnosis.
- HAM cocktail is highly effective for terminal restlessness.
- An adjustable hospital bed may be necessary for easing respiratory effort.
- Encourage the caregiver to process through one-on-one or in a group setting.

GINA

Life during the season of Covid had many twists and turns for everyone, especially the elderly. Gina was living in the city at an assisted living facility. Her granddaughter, Bea, lived in a smaller community nearby. This ALF looked pretty on the outside, and that was about it!

Gina was on Medicaid, and there was always potential for a roommate. One day, that happened, and things went downhill even more. The food was horrible, and the level of care was even worse. Often, she would press her call button, and no one would come. One day, Bea had to call 911 to come and help Gina.

The roommate would use the toilet, and it would not be cleaned up. Soiled adult briefs would not be thrown away properly. Bea's final straw was when she visited and brought her children. The roommate tested positive for Covid, and they tested Gina but did not tell Bea. That was it! She couldn't allow her precious grandmother to live in a place where the care was sub-par.

Bea took Gina to her cardiac appointment. She had been complaining of bloating in her belly, so the cardiologist made a referral to the GI doctor, who ordered a colonoscopy. During the procedure, they had to stop as she had a large mass in the colon, and they couldn't proceed. The results were positive for colon cancer. They offered her treatment and a colostomy bag.

With authority, 88-year-old Gina exclaimed, "I'm not going to *shit* in a bag!" Bea took her back to the assisted living facility.

At the time, Bea lived in a more rural area in her parent's two-story home and was contemplating buying the house. She told her husband she couldn't let her grandma die in that horrible ALF. The housing market was not very generous at the time.

Miraculously, they quickly found a ranch-style home in town that would be a better setup for caring for Gina. Even though it was more than they had budgeted, they had to move speedily. They closed on the house, and two days later, Bea brought Gina to live with her family. It was now six weeks after the official diagnosis of colon cancer. Gina was on hospice in the city, so we transitioned her care to our location.

Three months before Waylen moved in for his final days, Bea welcomed Gina, her grandmother, into her home. Bea's relationship with her grandmother was very special as she helped raise her and her sister. She had fond memories of being with Gina before and after school. Growing up, they loved to eat her quesadillas, which Gina coined, "cheese hickeys." To this day, that's what they were called in Bea's home.

It was very important to Bea for her five-year-old son to have some fond memories of his great-grandmother. Everyone living under one roof would allow for the creation of memories for the future. Bea just needed time.

I had a strong feeling that Gina instilled the Good Samaritan's values into Bea when she was a little toddler, unbeknownst to her. Enthusiasm, using your voice, and celebrating family were characteristics that surrounded Bea. This was nurtured and role-modeled to her by her loving grandma, Gina.

According to Bea, Gina was a spontaneous person who would get bored easily. She liked adventure, and, in general, she tended to be an anxious person. My first meeting with Gina was at the kitchen table. She had been in her new home for one week, and I took over for another case manager as we needed to alter some patients for locations.

Gina gingerly strolled out of the bedroom with her walker. I recalled her hair was all set and in place, and she was already dressed for the day. I noticed immediately that her hands were shaky with tremors, but she was in charge of the walker, and she maneuvered it with confidence.

Bea brought me the "medication tote" and laid it on the table. A very *large* tote, I might add! Out came many meds, and I mean many medications. There was a two-week bubble pack from the previous pharmacy, and then there were a few new meds, so I sorted the med box since our pharmacy didn't use the "bubble pack" system.

I brought a med list which did help, a little. I reviewed the meds with Gina, and we discussed her anxiety. It was very clear anxiety was her number one symptom. I placed the Xanax in the med box to be taken three times a day and then Lorazepam at bedtime to help with sleep. She didn't complain of pain in her abdomen. However, there were issues with constipation. I thought our first visit went well.

Later that afternoon, Bea called and was alarmed at what she saw when she helped Gina to the bathroom and was helping her wipe after a bowel movement. I came back and assessed the situation and took a picture to send to the medical director. I wasn't sure if I was seeing an enlarged hemorrhoid or a tumor starting to protrude from the rectum.

Our medical director said it could be a thrombosis hemorrhoid or rectal mass and to use hemorrhoid suppositories for one week and then reassess. Gina stated emphatically, "These hemorrhoids have been bothering me for a couple of years now!" Her abdomen was also starting to increase in circumference and getting more firm.

After a few days of using the suppositories, the bulge was becoming less in size. Still, it did have intermittent bleeding, so most likely, it was a thrombosis hemorrhoid. However, it had been three days with no bowel movement with senna two times a day, so sorbitol liquid was added to the regimen.

I gave Gina a bisacodyl suppository, and that did help her have a small bowel movement. She was still eating small portions three times a day and using her walker with minimal guidance. Her vital signs were all stable, and she did not need oxygen. She was having neck pain and using lidocaine patches and scheduled Tylenol for arthritis.

During our visit, Gina said she missed her husband and was ready to be with the Lord and him. Her husband died six months prior. Bea noticed the depression set in right after he passed as she started to lose the will to live. It is important to pay attention to your patient when they start talking about their deceased loved ones, as this marks the beginning of their readiness to transition.

Bea was struggling with the decision to take a work trip for five days. I explained that Gina was steady in her symptoms and vital signs at present. She was still eating, drinking, and ambulating with her walker. But you never know if things could change quickly. Sometimes, people choose to make their departure according to their timeline.

It was Thursday, and Bea's sister, Tonya, came in to help as Bea decided to go on the work trip. Gina had a rough night of pain in her stomach area. The scheduled Tylenol was more for the arthritis pain, so she tried her first dose of morphine at 0.25 ml with good relief, so a schedule was started for every six hours. As we were headed into the weekend, I requested another bottle of morphine, two Fentanyl patches, and a Yonker's suction machine.

Bea was out of town, and Gina was preparing for her transition. I called Bea with the update and said we would keep her informed. It was hard to imagine on day one of these symptoms the speed and trajectory of her decline that would occur.

That night, Tonya called the on-call nurse to make a visit. Gina was having more pain and anxiety, so the nurse administered morphine and Ativan. Her blood pressure was 70/40, and she was minimally responsive with O2 sats at 88% on room air. And just that quickly, Gina was in the active dying process. The on-call nurse left after she was settled, but Tonya called her to come right back as she started to have gurgles in her throat. The nurse readjusted her in bed and applied the Scopolamine patch.

The next day, I came to visit, and it took 2 ½ hours to get her symptoms better managed. Gina's abdomen was more swollen and taut than usual. A small amount of bowel movement was cleaned up. I placed the Foley catheter, and 400 ml of urine returned. After inserting the Macey catheter and giving Ativan and morphine, she was still uncomfortable, so I removed the Macey and did a digital to see if she was blocked higher up in the rectal vault.

That was affirmative. Bowel movement started to come out slowly after an enema. It was almost one hour of continuous slow movements and cleaning her up during the process. She was able to take Xanax, Ativan, and morphine orally during all of this.

I applied a Fentanyl patch as well to get that going. Finally, I was able to reinsert the Macey catheter, gave a dose of liquid morphine, and flushed it with 3 ml of water. The size of her abdomen had reduced after all the stool had been emptied; however, it was still increased in girth.

Gina was starting to calm down now and rest. I offered spiritual support, and she readily agreed to a prayer. I encouraged her to release from her body when she felt ready to transition. She said she wanted to go.

When I left, her oxygen saturation level was at 83%, and her knees were cold and mottled. Tonya lit a candle for soft light in her room and played her favorite hymns. I called Bea with an update as she was trying to get a flight back, but none were available until Monday.

The next day, when I arrived, Gina was in a deep coma. At times throughout the previous night, Tonya said she could hear her mumbling words but couldn't understand who she was talking to. I spoke with Bea, who was on the East Coast, and tried to encourage her not to feel guilty about going on the work trip.

I explained there is a choice when people want to make their transition. Knowing how close Gina and Bea were, it doesn't surprise me that she wanted to spare Bea the emotion of her departure. Gina died peacefully early the next morning, very well cared for in her granddaughter's home surrounded by loved ones.

The word hospice derives from the Latin word *Hospitum*, meaning hospitality or place of rest and protection for the ill and weary. Bea's delivery of hospitality was all-inclusive. She bestowed love and kindness by taking in her loved ones, whether they were biological family or not. She housed, fed, clothed, washed, and cared for them at every level possible. She helped in times of trouble and devoted herself to all kinds of good deeds. She was beautifully clothed in compassion, gentleness, and patience. *We need more Bea's in this world.*

Hospice Highlights

- Macy catheter is very effective with GI/Colon cancers, once fully cleared of bowel in the lower tract.
- Listen to your patient's whispers of their longing to go home and be with their loved ones.
- Choosing when they depart from their body is the last decision they ever get to make in this earthly realm.
- Embrace the experience as a provider when you get to connect with the Good Samaritan.

MY VET

Jay was a colorful man, and I knew that for his story, I would need to interview him as he had a way with words, eloquence, and humor that I needed to capture in a comprehensive atmosphere. Jay had lived seven decades and had a library of information inside him. Over 21 months on hospice service, he educated me on Vietnam, coming home after the war, cannabis use, and all its benefits, which you will see unfold in his story. I looked forward to every visit with Jay and his devoted home health caregiver, Zara.

I experienced a traumatic burn injury to a large portion of my body while camping. The doctors wanted to send me out of state for treatment. I refused to go as I would have no support system there. The VA found me a doctor, and he demanded I make a contract with him which stated, 'I don't quit on you, and you don't quit on me!' Every day, I had to get up and scrub my burns until they were clean. Mentally and physically, I quit. It hurt so bad; it was always on my mind. This treatment lasted five months for second and third-degree burns, which covered 70% of my body.

Then came the diagnosis around age 60 with anal cancer, and I decided to turn the reins over to the doctor. I had surgery and radiation for several months and endured severe nausea and weight loss. I told the doctor after all this, 'I quit, no more!'

The doctors told me I was in remission after the first round, but they also wanted me to do chemotherapy to seal the deal. I said, "I won't do chemotherapy because everyone I knew who did that died, and I'm already losing so much weight as it is after the radiation. They made me ring a bell!

In the Navy, if you flunk out, you ring a bell! In my mind, I flunked out. It's hard to imagine what that means when your strength and bigness define you. All my jobs required me to be big and strong; when they took that away, I didn't have anything.

Time travel back now to the early 2000s. I've had pain most of my life due to broken stuff and chronic pain from injuries. I could do the work of two men. Longshoreman was a high-risk job, and those were the kinds of jobs I went for.

After getting shot at in your life, back in Nam, you need something with a little thrill in it to keep you going!

During one of the parties with the biker gang, my girlfriend at the time grabbed my bottle of pain pills. When she put the pills down, she reached back in her hand with a 9-millimeter. As I reached for the gun, I took a few hits to my body and hips.

She shot me seven times. She was trying to get my Oxy, and I wasn't going to let that happen. After several years of being on Oxycontin, lawsuits came against them, and I was no longer prescribed this pain pill.

I had to look for something else to help manage my chronic pain. I smoked a lot of weed, and I noticed when I smoked the very strong kind, it helped the neuropathy pain. Now, I use it mostly in vape form, so other people around me won't be affected by it. At this point, I go through two cartridges per week, and with my Veteran's discount, it costs about $600.00 per month. Along with pain relief, I believe marijuana has slowed the progression of my disease. I think it's part of why I went into remission the first time because I started smoking a lot more dope right away.

You get a little scared, and then after that, you get mad, and then you don't freaking care. Was I gonna sit around and whine and cry about a date in the future? I came to a place where I accepted it. I just know my date will come sooner than yours!

It's a bad feeling to realize that you are mortal. Before I played the strong and big card, I thought I was invincible. When everything fell apart, I had to face up to my mortality. I thought I was way above that!

I wanted to know more about Jay's spiritual belief system and what brought him into that realm. So, I asked him about it.

I started engaging in Norse practice when I was in my 40s. I was having a hard time keeping my life together. You listen to one group that says you are a brave warrior, and another group says you are a worthless piece of nothing. I couldn't deal with that!

I didn't like the Christian religious groups. It probably had something to do with my dad, who was a preacher. He was very physically abusive to me in my childhood.

With Norse, they revered their warriors. They put them on a pedestal. Norse practice was mainly used to gain an edge during battle, to heal and draw strength from the gods. They were revered for what they did. They weren't persecuted. They were exonerated. When I got back from Vietnam I almost did myself in a few times. Who wants to be spit on and looked down upon?

It basically happened the first year I was back, but it never really quit. This is why a lot of guys did two and three tours, so they wouldn't have to come home.

Norse has many positive proverbs that kept me going in life. This was one of my favorites. 'Odin, father, let your light shine strong in my heart, fear of death; you alone have the might to heal, teach me to find Mimir's well between the dark forest threes teach me to cool my flames in the cool well of wisdom.'

Now that you have some background on Jay, I can tell his story. Upon admission, metastasis was present in the liver and mandible. There were no visible signs, such as jaundice or an enlarged abdomen. However, he did have a palpable area that was larger on one side of his jaw compared to the other.

Jay spent most of his time in his house watching TV or playing with his dog and treating his pain with MC (medical cannabis). In the early months, he would run errands with his caregiver a couple of times per week. However, the longstanding neuropathy in his feet affected his quality of life with poor mobility and pain.

He was on gabapentin for neuropathy and didn't want to increase his low dose. He was not a candidate for methadone, as he tried that once, and it gave him severe arrhythmia. He refused to use a cane even though he had several. He was a "frequent faller." I repeatedly encouraged him to use a cane or walker, but he admitted *his pride stood in the way*. Fortunately, he never sustained any major injuries with the falls.

As time progressed, the falls stopped, which is a very unusual element to see in a hospice patient's journey. The reality was hitting home, and Jay was too weak to get out for errands or mow his lawn on the riding lawn mower. He spent more time in his chair at home.

From the five to six-month mark, Jay's weight dropped 19 pounds. He woke up one morning and couldn't stop coughing and said he couldn't breathe. He thought he was going to die at that very moment! He quit smoking cigarettes cold turkey and never looked back. I recalled him telling me, "I'm not ready to die yet!"

His breakthrough use of morphine averaged three to four syringes of morphine at 0.5 ml daily. Since he was wearing his Fentanyl patch on his back, which was rather bony in appearance, I suggested we change the site of the Fentanyl to a fattier tissue area, like the abdomen, for better absorption. Within 12 hours, Jay was so somnolent he could hardly get out of bed. At the 48-hour mark, the patch was removed from the abdomen, and a new one was placed back on the usual site of his back. This was shocking as I've never seen anyone react this way to changing locations of the Fentanyl patch, especially to what is supposed to be the optimal way of efficacy for delivery.

A few months later, Jay wasn't using morphine at all, just a Fentanyl patch at 75 mcg. The nurse practitioner started him on MS Contin at 15 mg at nighttime so he could get through the night and not have to take morphine and interrupt his sleep cycle. This was a brilliant idea. We don't often mix narcotics like this with long-acting prescriptions, but in Jay's case, it worked.

After fifteen months on service, his pain started to escalate again, with morphine averaging three to four doses daily. The NP ordered 100 mcg of the Fentanyl patch, and he could not tolerate it. It made him sleep around the clock. So, back to 75 mcg, he stayed until the final weeks. With all the time in the recliner chair, a small stage two pressure injury developed. Wound care and applying the alternating pressure mattress to the chair helped keep this under control. It was my CNA's idea to put the air mattress on his recliner.

Jay was not ready for the hospital bed yet, as he said, "When that happens, I know I'm done!" The beauty of hospice is that it truly is a team effort to provide enrichment to the patient's life. The one thing Jay allowed our CNA to do for him was foot care every week. They had many a session of life review and colorful stories that he shared.

When our volunteer coordinator found out that Jay had never received a Quilt of Valor for his years of service in the military, she made that happen! She narrates the story, "Jay was sitting in his recliner while Zara was caring for him. I presented him with his Quilt of Valor and told him the story about the organization and how it was created. He cried tenderly while I thanked him for his service. He replied, 'Thank you for the support.' It was a very moving experience while I wrapped the beautiful quilt around his shoulders."

We also have a volunteer who calls our patients every Thursday to make sure all the supplies are in place for the weekend. When she discovered what Jay's favorite breakfast food was, she brought him biscuits and gravy one day. The tears in my strong vet's eyes at the delight of the southern treat reaffirmed to me the strength of our wonderful hospice team. One can never underestimate the beautiful acts of kindness shown to our patients and their impact on their lives.

Jay continued enjoying every day even though he was bound to his house. The relationship with his caregiver, Zara, was a beautiful thing to witness. The VA benefits of 30 plus hours per week for caregiver support were essential to continue his quality of life. He trusted Zara with the daily routine.

When I came back to work after being off for almost four months from the leg injury, the first thing I observed when I saw Jay was that global jaundice was visible. His abdomen was not distended. He had lost another ten pounds and needed help with all personal care except for eating. Upper respiratory symptoms presented and were managed with Sudafed and nebulizer treatments. After the second round of URI, Jay became oxygen-dependent. Sleeping increased to 18 plus hours per day.

Negotiations for the hospital bed began. After two weeks, it was placed in the living room so he would be in the center of all the activity.

At first, Jay would only take naps in it. He had to get used to it first. He knew in his heart once he got in it, he would make his journey.

His pain increased again. This time, a small titration was made with a 12 mcg Fentanyl patch added to the 75 mcg. He tolerated this well and was not over-sedated. As he slept more, the food intake decreased significantly, and it was time to move into the hospital bed so we could care for him with safety and ease.

Once he moved into the bed, he stopped eating. The pain increased as the cannabis use stopped. Jay averaged one ml of morphine every two hours and Ativan 0.4 ml every three hours for comfort in the final days. The Fentanyl was increased to 150 mcg at this point. Jay passed peacefully after 11 days of no food intake, surrounded by his family.

Jay encompassed a steadfast spirit with strength and perseverance throughout his hospice care for almost two years. I admired his tenacity and will to live for what each day would bring. I do believe that his use of cannabis was a significant component in relieving his pain. His symptoms were managed well with this choice of plan of care, and it played a role in his longevity.

Research is ongoing in Medical Cannabis use. "It demonstrates an overall to modest, long-term statistical improvement of all investigated measures including pain, associated symptoms and, importantly, reduction in opioid (and other analgesics) use."[23]

---

[23] PubMed Central, "The Effectiveness and Safety of Medical Cannabis for Treating Cancer-Related Symptoms in Oncology Patients," 2024, https://www.ncbi.nlm.nih.gov/pmc/articles/PMC9163497/.

Hospice Highlights

- Document teaching and education for fall prevention.
- Observe how the patient's body responds to titrations in narcotics and make adjustments accordingly.
- Medical Cannabis is an adjunctive to treating cancer pain.

Source

23) PubMed Central. "The Effectiveness and Safety of Medical Cannabis for Treating Cancer-Related Symptoms in Oncology Patients." https://www.ncbi.nlm.nih.gov/pmc/articles/PMC9163497/.

LIFE REVIEW

I had been given a verbal report on Joe but wasn't sure what to expect when I first met him. This was my first experience taking care of someone with the diagnosis of inclusion body myositis. Inclusion body myositis is a rare muscle inflammatory disease that affects only 20,000 people in the USA, usually men over 50.[24]

IBM causes muscle weakness and degeneration in specific regions of the body. The wrists, fingers, front of the thighs, and front of the legs below the knee are the most common sites. It leads to severe wasting and weakness of the arm and leg muscles. People usually experience symptoms for five years before a diagnosis is made. Within 15 years of diagnosis, the loss of mobility and strength leads to full dependence with ADLs (activities of daily living) and often becoming bedbound. IBM is often classified as an indirect cause of death due to dysphagia, aspiration pneumonia, and respiratory failure.[25]

When I saw Joe lying in his hospital bed, I envisioned him riding on a motorcycle back in the day. He fit the profile! A strong-willed, burly man dressed in black leather venturing on the highway. His favorite apparel was a white t-shirt and hair braided in a thin

---

[24] MDA Quest, "Simply Stated: Inclusion Body Myositis Revisited," https://mdaquest.org/simply-stated-inclusion-body-myositis-revisited/.

[25] MDA, "Inclusion Body Myositis," https://www.mda.org/disease/inclusion-body-myositis.

ponytail with sheets and blankets tucked to his sides to keep his cold hands warm. Sally, his bride, was thankful to have hospice's help as she had grown weary over the past several months of multiple trips to the hospital.

When the hospice informational process was done in the hospital setting, Joe said he was done with treatments and was ready to stop using the Trilogy ventilator. He was prepared to transition to the oxygen concentrator for comfort measures. But, after his first week at home, Joe began having second thoughts about stopping using the ventilator. He was not ready to quit fighting the disease he had lived with for ten years.

This was not Joe's decision to make alone. Sally had stood by his side as his primary caregiver and devoted wife. She was desperately in need of support to help care for Joe. Sally could not do this by herself any longer. She was suffering from caregiver burnout. Joe was completely bedbound. He had no use of his hands or legs. His hands pointed downward and inward in a contracted position. His circulation was poor, and his hands were often dusky blue, cold, and edematous. Two years prior, he had a heart attack and stroke, which triggered the downward spiral of events leading to bedbound status.

I remember driving home late in the afternoon when Sally called me and said they were ready to discuss things in more detail. She wanted me to reiterate the benefits of hospice support and the importance of the ventilator at this juncture in his prognosis. I will not forget that conversation, as Sally prepared her questions well, which helped Joe understand what I explained.

I clarified to Joe that the support he would receive for his disease process was not only in the form of oxygen but also the narcotic management that he required for the past several years. Managing the long-acting pain medications along with the air rescue benefit of liquid morphine would become his good friend in the weeks ahead. He would also have liquid Ativan to help with the anxiety component. I placed more emphasis on medication management versus oxygen. Nursing visits would be three times a week, with aide support, chaplain, social work, and volunteer assistance. It is extremely important that we be there to support Sally and help her through this emotional and spiritual process.

I was so proud of Sally as she spoke up for herself in the conversation. She told Joe she could not do this alone any longer. The frequent trips to the hospital were not a good quality of life, and she needed help from the hospice team in their home. The conversation closed as they needed time to think about it. Sally called me back 20 minutes later and said they would stay with hospice and give up using the Trilogy ventilator. And so, the journey began.

Technically, Joe's admitting diagnosis was chronic respiratory failure with hypercapnia, but it was the inclusion body myositis that brought him to the place of terminal illness. His comorbidities included hypertensive heart disease with heart failure, atrial fibrillation, chronic pain, and dysphagia. Joe used oxygen during the day as needed and routinely at night. The absence of the Trilogy ventilator was not a traumatic change in his plan of care. I believe this was because we worked with Joe on proper pain management and symptom management for anxiety associated with air hunger.

According to Sally, Joe had a colorful past. We didn't get into all the details, but she briefly mentioned drug addiction decades prior. Joe was on 100 mg of MS Contin two times a day at the start of care. He took immediate-release morphine tablets for breakthrough pain. The adjectives he used to describe his pain were burning, sharp, and deep. These were neuropathic pain descriptors to a T.

He was on a few medications to help with this, but they were at entry levels of dosage and ineffective. The Nortriptyline was at 25 mg at bedtime, and gabapentin 100 mg twice a day. Both medications take weeks to build in levels of therapeutic support.

Joe also needed to be on methadone. We started the educational process on what methadone was and how it helped neuropathy pain tremendously. Joe was extremely leery about switching from MS Contin to methadone. He had been on this routine for several years and didn't believe me when I told him how it had helped several of my patients over the years. I brought up the discussion weekly.

Finally, after eight weeks, he decided to give it a try. The NP started him on 0.5 ml (5 mg) two times a day. Three days later, there was no improvement, so the NP ordered 1 ml (10 mg) two times a day. He weaned off the MS Contin over one week, and it was a smooth transition. The neuropathy pain in his legs finally began to experience relief!

The five big symptom issues Joe experienced were pain, air hunger, anxiety, constipation, and dysphagia. I reassured Joe and Sally that they wouldn't run out of liquid morphine and Ativan. Teaching was done about the disease process at almost every visit, and that as the body declined, it needed more medication. This was normal.

Joe averaged taking 1 ml of morphine four to five times per day. Ativan in liquid form 2 mg/ml started at a dose of 0.3 ml. This medication helped with anxiety, but it made him extra sleepy at first. Over time, he titrated up to 1 ml dosage.

The breakthrough doses of morphine averaged four to five times per day. The protocol would be to increase the long-acting methadone to 1 ml three times a day. The reason Joe took morphine so frequently was mostly for the symptom of air hunger. It did alleviate this for 3-hour segments on average. It also helped with the breakthrough pain, but not entirely, as the pain was neuropathic.

After several rounds of negotiation, Joe and I agreed on the bowel protocol. He could be a little bit stubborn at times, but then I could be quite persistent. If there was no movement by day three, I would give an enema. He was on several stool softeners, including four Senna S per day. We then tried liquid Sorbitol.

That was a big mistake, as the texture of the liquid triggered his dysphagia, and he had a huge choking and coughing spell that lasted for an hour. We used the Yonkers suction machine and Ativan to help recover from that. Needless to say, he never wanted that medication ever again. Within the week, he started on a Scopolamine patch to help with secretions, and soon after, Atropine drops were added.

To enhance the bowel regimen, bisacodyl tabs were added, 10 mg every morning. I encouraged Sally to add more fiber to his diet with ground flax. She started to put this in the sweet treats she would bake. Since it was hidden in the treats, Joe couldn't taste it, which was important because he was a meat and potatoes man. Joe lacked muscle strength due to the IBM, so enemas became a ritual, usually two times per week. The last few weeks before he stopped eating, he required digital removal as well. There was no ability to evacuate on his own.

Establishing trust with this couple was vital to prove that the hospice team would be there for them. It was not just nursing and certified nursing assistant support; they also had a wonderful volunteer. It took Sally three weeks to accept this help. The volunteer would sit with Joe while Sally would go out for a few hours to have lunch with a friend or to run errands. This helped the caregiver burnout she had been experiencing. Their priest would also make routine visits, and our chaplain supported them.

Every week involved teaching Sally about the disease process and what was occurring throughout Joe's body while he was slowly declining. Providing an ear to listen to her concerns and anxiety about the dying process was a part of almost every visit. Joe had the Foley catheter placed at the previous hospitalization before hospice admission. It was essential to stay in for comfort measures as turning Joe for brief changes was challenging due to his size and inability to use his arms.

One of the symptoms of ongoing concern for Sally was the sediment and color changes in the urine that occurred over the three months Joe was on hospice. To address the functionality of the catheter, I did bag changes about every three weeks. Our medical director emphasized comfort rather than routine monthly change out of the entire catheter, as this could introduce new bacteria. Bacteriuria is the presence of bacteria in urine. The incidence of bacteriuria is 3 to 7% per day. After one month duration of an indwelling Foley catheter, nearly 100% of patients will have bacteriuria.[26]

Sally had concerns that an infection was developing. I focused on explaining that colonization of bacteria happens after one month, which is normal for an indwelling catheter. It was not causing pain or burning, and the urine flowed well with bag changes. Antibiotics were not necessary. It didn't require flushing with normal saline, either. Explaining symptomology in practical terms is vital, as families can sometimes go to other sources for advice.

Six weeks before Joe transcended, he had an incident where his oxygen saturation levels dropped into the 80s while on oxygen at

---

[26] Centers for Disease Control and Prevention, "Indwelling Urinary Catheters," https://www.cdc.gov/hai/prevent/cauti/indwelling/overview.html.

four liters. Sally's anxiety escalated, so I placed him on daily visits. I thought Joe was possibly around three weeks from passing, but that was not the case. This event coincided with the deep inward processing work that Joe needed to go through on many levels. Up to this point, his mantra had been, "I'm not ready to die yet. I'm going to keep living."

We were experiencing some mild windstorms during this winter, around 50 to 60 mph. The wind, along with 10 inches plus of snow, caused several power outages in Joe's neighborhood. Since he was on four liters of oxygen, the backup E tank would only last a couple of hours with the electricity out. We couldn't supply him with 8 or 10 E tanks per storm. It wasn't feasible, as these storms were happening back-to-back.

The power outages lasted 24 hours and sometimes even longer. We negotiated a plan to go to two liters on the oxygen, and he would supplement with morphine or Ativan if the air hunger became severe. This way, he could get longer use out of the E tank when the power went out. His other option was to have a respite stay at our contracted facility. That was a hard no. Joe said he did not want to leave his house.

Joe began to see his deceased mom in the room and started talking to her. Then the life review conversations began with him mumbling under his breath while he slept. Sometimes, you could clearly understand what Joe was saying, and other times, you could not. This alarmed Sally at first, but I reassured her this was normal and he had to do this inner soul work.

When the talk became unintelligible, Sally felt the hallucinations needed to be addressed. So, the nurse practitioner ordered haloperidol. After one dose, Sally believed the hallucinations were getting worse, so she didn't want to give haloperidol anymore. He remained on Ativan for the anxiety with more frequent dosing with an increase in mg amount, which did help alleviate this symptom. Joe's food intake gradually declined. He stopped eating 12 days before he crossed over, except for a few sips of fluid the last few days.

As we neared the end of Joe's journey, Sally hoped his brother would visit one more time. We talked with his brother, Mark, on speakerphone and gave him the update. Mark was on a plane two days later and visited for a week. This was a critical piece of Joe's final days. Sally was in tune with the need for this integral part of the dying process and gently pushed to make it happen.

During this time, the family reached out to other siblings where communication had not existed for over a decade. One cannot underestimate the necessity of live review and closure with family members. I believe that the patient will linger in the dying process if life review is not encouraged or dismissed as random hallucinations.

Five themes may be experienced in the life review process: expression, responsibility, forgiveness, acceptance, and gratitude. Joe's expression of emotion during these months was largely one of bargaining. He wanted more time; he was not ready to die. He wasn't angry, just not ready.

Joe began recounting his life stories in his mind and tried to express them verbally. A realization occurs that you have played a role in everything that has happened to you in life; this is called responsibility. He was a devout believer in the Catholic faith. He understood and had received forgiveness. Acceptance came after time spent with his brother and the family phone calls. In my heart, I believe Joe felt gratitude when he chose to depart this earth on his favorite holiday, Thanksgiving. Joe died with a spirit of peace in his heart, with his beautiful bride at his side.

Hospice Highlights

- Be patient and allow time to begin more efficient pain medication management.
- Manage bacteriuria with Foley bag changes or normal saline flushes. Antibiotics are not always the answer.
- The life review process includes expression, responsibility, forgiveness, acceptance, and gratitude.

Source

24) MDA Quest, "Simply Stated: Inclusion Body Myositis Revisited," https://mdaquest.org/simply-stated-inclusion-body-myositis-revisited/
25) MDA. "Inclusion Body Myositis." https://www.mda.org/disease/inclusion-body-myositis
26) CDC. "Indwelling Urinary Catheters." www.cdc.gov/hai/prevent/cauti/indwelling/overview.html.

EXCENTRIC EXIT

This story was not my firsthand experience to share but rather one of my amazing co-workers, Denise. In all my years as a hospice nurse in the great land of Alaska, I never encountered a scenario like this.

Hazel and her husband, James, lived in a very remote area about 40 miles from town. This location was considered off-grid, but fortunately, it had electricity. They had lived in this setting for four decades and enjoyed an independent lifestyle far removed from city life and the intrusion of people. Denise described a peaceful setting next to a pristine lake with snow-capped mountain views and no other houses in sight.

We were fast approaching the season of Breakup, what lower 48 folks would call Spring. The lake was still covered with copious amounts of snow and deep layers of ice. This year, a record snowfall of over 130 inches occurred. The temperatures would rise to 40 degrees in the daytime but then go back down to below freezing at night.

This pattern repeated itself for several weeks as temperatures gradually rose to encourage the snow to vanish and allow greenery to appear. But first must come the mud. Brown, messy earth incorporated into every aspect of our lives for several weeks until summer would magically appear.

The final portion of the journey to get to their cabin involved a road that was termed a 'forestry-cleared road.' In rural Alaska, this typically meant a road that was constructed through a forested area, allowing access to remote regions. Denise depicted the road as narrow, basically wide enough for one vehicle to drive on, and it was not maintained in any way, shape, or form. It had bumps, ridges, and ruts, Alaska at its finest.

When Hazel came on to hospice service, there was apprehension from multiple team members about how we would get to the destination since we were almost in Breakup season. In emergency situations, the on-call nurse would need to make visits in a timely fashion. Would this be possible?

James had offered to pick up the nurse in his 4-wheeler and drive the 1.5-mile road to their home. Denise expressed safety concerns about his ability to drive with another passenger on board. Would she fall off and get hurt, or would they get stuck in the mud? Was this a regular 4-wheeler or a side-by-side with seatbelts?

A couple of other team members offered to do visits if needed. I was uncomfortable helping as memories of a side-by-side incident of me falling out and down a hill and hitting my head on a tree still haunted me. That was a near-death experience I did not want to repeat! I could not risk activities that would engage potentially broken bones at this point in my life after the previous year's leg injury. At least side-by-sides had seatbelts, but they can be topsy-turvy in their mobility. It didn't take much for them to tip over, especially if the surface was sketchy!

Hazel had been experiencing spontaneous vomiting with any food but no nausea or abdominal pain. Over the past several months, she had lost 20 pounds. With extensive activity, she would get lightheaded and pass out. She said these symptoms mimicked what happened previously when she had a nasal obstruction and subsequently underwent a nasal polypectomy/sinuplasty. She had COPD and was a current smoker.

Hazel went to her primary doctor, and the CT scan results revealed a pleural effusion with right lung atelectasis and a very large mass in the right lung. The adrenal glands showed bilateral masses and peritoneal nodules, indicating peritoneal metastasis. When Hazel heard the news, she adamantly told her doctor that she did not want further investigation or interventions. She understood she would die and wanted hospice to support her for the end of life.

EXCENTRIC EXIT

Hazel was matter-of-fact in her approach to the diagnosis, just as she had been over the course of 40 years, living a life of self-reliance and hard work. She would carry these attributes into her final weeks of life. Remember, people die in the manner of how they have lived their lives. Characteristics and personality traits do not change suddenly.

Denise's first visit with Hazel and James was possible with her SUV. The forestry cleared road was still frozen and passable. Hazel sat on her couch and went through the necessary motions of interaction with Denise. Hazel asked, "What will we do with all this equipment?" She didn't think there would be a need for oxygen. Denise explained she might want to use the oxygen as needed if the shortness of breath became more severe. Hazel remained distant.

Vital signs and a discussion on pain and other symptoms ensued. Hazel was very clear with Denise that she didn't want any medications and no pull-ups or chux pads! She didn't even want the comfort pack with emergency medications, but Denise insisted, as this was our policy. We had to have meds in the house ready for various emergencies that might arise to keep her comfortable.

Denise asked Hazel if our nurses couldn't reach her cabin due to the road conditions, would she consider staying in town for the time being. Both Hazel and James quickly refuted that idea. They were adamant they would stay on their own property and home.

During the following week, Denise insisted on the bedside commode so Hazel wouldn't have to walk 40 feet from her living room area (which is where she resided) to the bathroom. She thought this would help with the exacerbation of air hunger and the energy required to walk to the bathroom multiple times throughout the day and night.

The equipment company delivered the bedside commode to the end of the driveway. James took it from there and strapped it to the 4-wheeler to get it to the cabin. Hazel didn't use this, not even one time! She said, "This is one thing that I can hold on to doing."

She was willing to use the nebulizer with ipratropium and albuterol combination to help with her breathing and air hunger, but not the oxygen. During every visit, Denise would try to educate them about the dying process and ask if they had any questions. Hazel was always silent and expressed no concern about the process.

Oxygenation levels slowly started to decline, and she presented with a baseline of unawareness of the elements transpiring. Most likely, Hazel was retaining Co_2, and confusion was starting to settle in. Denise recalled, "They were such independent Alaskans, you just don't mess with strong, self-determined Alaskan women! I think they each had their role, and James respected that, honored her, and let her carry on that role."

After ten days on service, Hazel was ready to start using the morphine. James didn't think it was odd that Hazel used morphine in a manner in which she had not been instructed to do so. She put it in her nebulizer to breathe it in versus taking it orally as prescribed. When Denise saw what she had been doing, she explained the morphine was meant to be taken orally and showed them both what the dosage ranges were along with the written medication list.

Hazel wanted minimal intervention from the hospice team. The following week, Hazel was using low-dose morphine orally multiple times per day. She needed help walking to the bathroom and toilet and then back to the couch.

The next week, Denise called the morning of her scheduled visit to see what time would be good and if they needed any supplies. James declined and said, "They didn't need a visit." He then called Denise in the afternoon and said, "I think her eyes are fluttering, but she isn't responding or talking. Denise asked, "Have you tried to wake her up?" James said, "No." Denise called our supervisor and was instructed to visit to assess the situation.

James met Denise at the end of the driveway at 3 pm. She was cloaked in all her outdoor apparel: overalls, gloves, mud boots and helmet. It was an exciting mud fest of travelling about 10 mph over the *forestry cleared road* that was laden with bumps and puddles. By the time they got to the cabin Denise was completely covered in mud from head to toe. She was proud of herself for making the journey and that James was a safe chauffeur. After taking all external gear off before entering the cabin, with one glance to the living room, it was obvious that Hazel had passed. Hazel was motionless and sitting partially upright on her couch but slumped to the right side. She was extremely stiff as rigor mortis had set in. She most likely had passed about 12 hours prior.

Denise listened for a heartbeat and confirmed that Hazel had died. James didn't respond with tears or emotion. He just stood there and watched. Since Hazel had declined any briefs or incontinence supplies, there was nothing to put under her for protection. James found some Visqueen from his garage and cut a portion so Denise could put it under Hazel while her body lay on the couch.

Stoically, James said he needed time to set up the transport as he had to borrow the trailer from his neighbor. James told Denise that she didn't need to come back the next morning to help get her out. He could do it himself. Denise asked if he had anyone to help him, and he replied, "No, I can do it by myself."

Denise envisioned poor Hazel being wrapped up in a tarp, dragged out of the house, and winched onto a trailer. Denise emphatically said, "I will be back in the morning to help you." James didn't argue with Denise.

The next morning, James picked Denise up at 7 am on the 4-wheeler. They wrapped Hazel in a blanket, and surprisingly, a family member showed up to help carry her to the trailer. They laid her on the tarp, covered her with it, and secured her tightly with ratchet straps to the trailer.

This time, James drove even more slowly over the 1.5-mile road. About 100 feet from the road, two moose casually glanced at the activity while foraging for food and then returned to eating their breakfast. They didn't disrupt Hazel's departure.

The plan was made for an 8 am meeting of the funeral home at the end of the driveway. They had backed up to the driveway and were prepared. It was critical to transport her at this early hour while the road was still frozen so they wouldn't get stuck in the ruts. Can you imagine Hazel's final journey if that would have happened?

They transferred Hazel into the funeral home SUV. Up until this point, James had shown no emotion whatsoever. He was reserved in his mannerism. As they went to load her in the vehicle, he finally broke down, cried, and gave her a hug. He thanked her for everything she did to help them. This was an adventure Denise would never forget!

Hospice Highlights

- People die in the manner they have lived their lives. Don't expect to change this.
- Be brave, safe, and use wisdom for all methods of transportation involved in traveling to your patient and assisting in their transport.

ONCE UPON A STORYTIME

This story takes place in 1996, in sunny Florida, where my grandparents resided for their retirement years. They lived in a double-wide trailer park community for people over 55. I have fond memories as a teenager in the 1980s, visiting them for weeks at a time during the summer. It was a delight to go on an extended vacation from Alaska to Florida as a teen.

Gigi, my grandmother, loved hospitality, parties, dining out, and shopping and was very much a gift giver. She passed on to my sister and me a love for precious, beautiful China and the stories that went with each dish. This was a unique way of continuing memories of our ancestors, great-grandparents, and beyond. Poppop, my grandfather, loved the beach. We spent countless hours by the waves soaking up the sun, applying coconut-scented sunscreen, and simply relaxing and swimming. They were both very devoted and loving grandparents even though thousands of miles separated us physically.

A unique thing happened during my recovery from the broken leg in 2023, allowing me time to complete this book project. One of my nurse-mates came to visit me bearing gifts. She presented me with a book with a special inscription. "To Esther Pepper from Gigi, 1979. The gentleman who walked your mom down the aisle when she married your dad gave each of you kids a copy of this book. This is the last one that I had. Love Gigi."

How in the world did she have this book titled *Once Upon a Storytime*? It was an elementary reader, hardback, with fun illustrations in color and in black and white. Somehow, this book went from my house to someone's house in the family and on to Goodwill many years ago. I never would have parted with it. I saved all of my letters from Gigi over the years.

My friend was going through her book collection when she saw the inscription and knew it was meant to come back to me. This special surprise clarified that this chapter's title would be *Once Upon a Storytime*. This story about Gigi is the foundation of why I am writing this book. Isn't it amazing how surprising events can happen and bring things back full circle?

In early 1996, Gigi was diagnosed with non-Hodgkin's lymphoma at age 75. She chose aggressive treatment with chemotherapy. Gigi did not want to die and was very fearful of the process. She would tell everyone close to her, "I want to live, I want to live!"

My grandmother was a third-generation person of strong faith. Even though she knew where she was going when she died, the process of going through the unknown caused her much apprehension. She expressed fear of not being able to breathe when the time came. Fears are real and need to be addressed, yet with that, we have to engage with the spiritual, mental, and emotional for help. Gigi was nervous by nature and suffered from chronic anxiety her entire life. A unique element of anxiety is its ability to imagine a negative future outcome.[27]

Her sister, my Great Aunt Ciel, was the complete opposite. During the second world war, both Poppop and my Great Uncle Al served their country in uniform. Poppop was in the Navy and based in the U.S. His job was to teach officers how to shoot machine guns. Uncle Al served as a rifleman and followed the tanks. He would never speak of those events and the duties he had to perform.

Aunt Ciel suffered from severe depression during this time, but after the war was over, she made a choice. Her countenance changed when Uncle Al came home. She never said negative things about anyone or any situation. She always tried to stay positive or listen. Her optimism was contagious! Sometimes, this would frustrate Gigi because she felt she wasn't being realistic. But both sisters loved each other immensely and had a beautiful faith.

---

[27] Psychology Today, "The Biology of Anxiety," https://www.psychologytoday.com/intl/basics/anxiety/the-biology-anxiety.

There are many studies that validate the power of words and how this affects our lives and those that we love. In the book *Words Can Change Your Brain*, Newburg and Waldman explain that "Negative words release stress and anxiety-inducing hormones. Negative words, whether they are spoken, heard, or thought, cause situational stress and contribute to long-term anxiety. Exercising positive thoughts can change one's reality."[28]

My dad shared some interesting thoughts as to why Gigi may have been anxious. He said it could be genetics or her heritage and what they left behind in Europe. On Gigi's side, our ancestors came to America, fleeing from the Anabaptists' persecution in Europe in the late 1800s.

During World War II, seeing the extermination of the Jews and many other racial groups elicited fear as they were afraid of what Hitler was doing. This included Hitler's radical thinking for many years before World War II. My father was nine years old when the family members all lived together to support each other financially and emotionally during this time.

One of Gigi's wishes was for her son to live across the street from her, "So I could see you through the window, and you could see me, and we would be close to each other." A beautiful blessing occurred in 1996 when the neighbors across the street from Poppop and Gigi offered their trailer to my parents so they could be close to help care for her over the following eight months. She finally got her wish to have her only child, her son, live next to her, even if it was just for a short time in her old age. This made her so happy.

I remember receiving the call from my parents in late September of 1996. I was working as an LPN at a nursing home at the time. My parents, Aunt Ciel, and Uncle Al had been taking turns being with her around the clock in the hospital for three weeks. They did not trust that she would be cared for properly if someone wasn't there 24/7. They were utterly exhausted.

My parents were in their mid-50s at the time, and they reached out to me because I was the only one of my siblings who could come

---

[28] Behavioral Research & Marketing Institute, "The Neuroscience Behind Words," https://brm.institute/neuroscience-behind-words/.

to help. Gigi was declining rapidly, and they knew she would be dying there and not going back home. My boss gave me a week off to go to Florida to be with my family. I was so thankful as it was such quick notice.

I was 25 years old and only one year into my nursing career. There were so many things yet to learn. I was a floor nurse administering medications and performing minor wound care in the nursing home. My interest in end-of-life care was taking root in this setting. Seeing residents being sent out to the hospital for their tune-up sessions for COPD and CHF only to go back to the nursing home and then a month later be sent out again. This cycle repeated itself over and over again.

I remember one patient would just sit there in her wheelchair crying and ask me, "Why do I have to go to the hospital again? I just want to be comfortable and die here. Why won't my family let me die? This is my home."

I wanted to be their advocate, helper, and voice to their family and the doctor to honor their wishes. The desire to be the patient's supporter and be vocal in this area came naturally to me. I'm not sure how, as I was more of an introvert and quiet in those early years. I recalled getting several patients onto hospice services in the nursing home. It was good to have extra support for patients and their families, and this ensured the residents stayed in their home setting and did not have to be in the sterile environment of the hospital to die.

Before my arrival, my parents informed me of the experience with Gigi in the hospital. They likened it to being in a third-world country. They initiated a plan for all four of the available adults to do 6-hour shifts by Gigi's side. She was never left alone. There were too many mistakes being made.

At shift change, the nurse had given the medication but didn't document it on the clipboard. Then, the next nurse came in to give the same medicine, and my dad stopped her, stating, "I just saw the other nurse give the same medication one hour ago." He started to record the conversations when the doctor visited.

Then, a most incomprehensible thing happened. The surgery techs came to get Gigi for surgery. She was semi-responsive, and it was obvious she was in the dying process. "What surgery?" my dad inquired. "We never agreed to any more procedures." The nurse responded, "But this is how we learn." He replied angrily, "You won't learn on my dying mother!"

Seeing Gigi lying in the hospital bed so frail, weighing around 110 pounds and actively dying, was surreal. Knowing that I would not be seeing her again for 50-plus years until it was my time to transcend was heart-wrenching.

A week prior, her lungs were starting to shut down, and the DNR order had not been written yet, so she received a chest tube. She had a non-rebreather mask on for extra airflow. She was in and out of consciousness and still fearful, so apparently, extra oxygen was standard at the time. She made eye contact upon my arrival, acknowledged that I was there, and squeezed my hand.

That first night with her, the night shift nurse was kind and would give her pain medication, morphine, when I asked. She was not on any schedule for pain or anxiety medication. We had to ask every single time. I asked the nurse why she couldn't be on a schedule for the pain medication, and the reply was, "She had to be showing signs of being in pain in order to receive the medication."

This made no sense. Shortness of breath and moaning in pain because your body is shutting down on top of being bedbound for three weeks elicits pain. Even my patients in the nursing home were on scheduled pain medications, those who had symptoms with ongoing disease processes. They didn't have to ask every time.

The following day, Gigi's symptoms escalated. Her breathing was more labored and irregular, and you could hear her crackly breathing. The IV fluids were running at a rate of 75 cc/hr. I asked the nurse why she had IV fluids going into her at such a high rate. Her response was "to keep her hydrated." Even with my limited knowledge at the time, I responded with, "You are making her lungs fill up with fluid faster as she's dying, and the rest of her body is increasing with edema in her legs and arms. This is not comforting to her."

When I would help the nurse reposition her in the bed, Gigi would moan in pain. I asked if she could have morphine, and the response was, "Her respirations are only eight per minute. She could stop breathing if I give her morphine." I begged her to call the doctor and get the order because she had the right to be comfortable while she was dying.

When she refused, I found the charge nurse and asked her to do so, and she did. An hour later, she received morphine as an intramuscular injection, not by mouth. They reduced the rate to 20 cc/hr on the IV fluid. What Gigi feared the most was actually happening; she was struggling to breathe at the very end.

I called my sister and brother so they could say their goodbyes over the phone. I wasn't sure of the significance of this at the time, as I had only seen a few people die in the nursing home. Those were difficult calls to make, but it felt like they were in the room with Gigi and me, and feeling their presence was special. This helped bring my siblings closure since they couldn't be physically present.

Then, the night nurse came in as it was day three, and the peripheral IV site needed to be changed. After three unsuccessful attempts at access, I asked her to please chart that the family refused for her to keep trying. The IV was finally discontinued. Everything on her plan of care was not geared towards dying with dignity and comfort. It was a battle every step of the way for Gigi to release and make her journey.

The next day, Gigi's respiratory pattern was Cheyne stokes with an automatic reflexive movement of her mouth and upper respiratory muscles. She was starting to mottle on her feet and was cooler to touch. That night, my dad was with me. He was sleeping in the chair. I woke him up because Gigi's respirations were slowly winding down like a clock now, eight, five, and then three per minute with long pauses in between.

I asked Dad if he wanted to read scripture to her. He read Psalm 23 and followed with more verses. Then, her breathing stopped at 3:33 am on October 3.

There is a choice in the matter of when the person is ready to leave the physical shell of their body. Gigi was a perfectionist. I smiled when I saw the time had to do with consecutive numbers of three. This was precise and reflected her passion for detail. Finally, she was at peace. No more anxiety, no more suffering with tubes in her body, and pain from the lymphoma. She was in the presence of the Lord and so many loved ones.

This experience solidified the future of my profession. I knew the direction my nursing career was heading. In my heart, I wanted to be an advocate for those who wanted peace, comfort, and dignity in their last days.

What my grandmother experienced in the hospital setting when she was actively dying overwhelmed me with tremendous grief. It broke my heart to see the lack of knowledge and understanding about the dying process and how comfort measures should honor someone who was truly in pain and suffering. I wanted to learn as much as I could about this specialty, so I went to gain a foundation in oncology and neurology in a large urban hospital setting.

For three years, I cared for those who received stem cell transplants, chemotherapy, radiation, and those who suffered from cerebral vascular accidents and other neurological disease processes. I developed many skills and experienced volumes in the fast-paced hospital setting. I learned the concept and beauty of team nursing as RNs were paired with LPNs. I earned my RN degree during this time.

The older nurses I worked with knew I was passionate about talking to families about end-of-life care. When their patients were at that place, they would come and get me to talk with the family to explain the symptoms they would be going through and support them. I was now ready to step into the world of hospice and experience what this word truly meant.

Hospice is derived from the Latin word *hospitum*, meaning hospitality. I hoped to bring honor to my Gigi, who loved being hospitable. I would endeavor to return that hospitable love to the terminally ill.

Hospice Highlights

- Hospice nurses must always advocate for their patients. Supporting their need for dying with respect, dignity, and comfort is a priority.
- Hospitality, demonstrating kindness and generosity, is at the heart of who we are and what we do.
- Hospital settings provide very different approaches in healthcare focused on attempting to improve the disease process. This can conflict with best practices for those who are in the dying process.

Source

27) Psychology Today. "The Biology of Anxiety." https://www.psychologytoday.com/intl/basics/anxiety/the-biology-anxiety
28) Behavioral Research & Marketing Institute. "The Neuroscience Behind Words." https://brm.institute/neuroscience-behind-words/

IN THE BEGINNING

Amazing events can happen when the body begins its journey to leave the physical and transcend to the spiritual realm. This particular story occurred in my first year at the nursing home. I literally had no clue that these scenarios took place. I had been working for a few months on the 3 to 11 p.m. shift. I was passing medications, and one of the CNAs came running down the hallway to get me as they were very alarmed at what Miss Grace was doing and saying.

Miss Grace had dementia and moderate agitation most of the time. Her words were repetitive when she spoke, and you could never understand her thought process. Her speech was nonsensical. She spent most of her days in her wheelchair, scooting up and down the hallways, rambling and agitated.

When I walked into the room, she was lying in her bed, looking upward toward the ceiling. Her body's countenance was one of complete peace. It was as if her soul was engaging with other beings in the room as if she were with them. Her speech was 100% clear and a little repetitive, but her words were precise. The following discourse occurred over a couple of hours.

Grace: Spelled the word m-o-t-h-e-r, m-o-t-h-e-r, repeatedly.
Me: Why are you spelling the word, mother?
Grace: Because she's calling me home. I haven't seen her in a long time.
Me: Are you in any pain?
Grace: No.

Me: Do you see a light?
Grace: Yes.
Me: What does it look like?
Grace: A big electric light.
Me: What is the light doing?
Grace: It is pulling me upward. (then I started to cry)
Me: What are you doing now?
Grace: I'm with my cousin. She's holding my hand in the light.
Me: Do you still see your mother?
Grace: No, not anymore.
Me: Do you know what the light is?
Grace: Jesus is so wonderful. I'm walking through a town.
Me: Are the people happy or sad?
Grace: Sad.

Some time passed, and Miss Grace started talking about the First National Bank. Then she rattled off some numbers to a street address for Caster Knotts and shopping.

Grace: I see three or four of them. (repeated several times)
Me: Three or four of what?
Grace: Three outlines, brothers and sisters.
Me: Are you afraid, Miss Grace?
Grace: Not now.
Me: Why not?
Grace: I've been approved by the light. A-p-p-r-o-v-a-l. (She spelled this word repeatedly for five minutes or so.)
Me: Is there anything you want to tell us?
Grace: You are too young to know.
Me: Know what?
Grace: To be approved by the light.
Me: What is the light doing now?
Grace: Walking towards the light. It is getting brighter. I'm being guided by the light. E-x-t-r-a light. I like the light. The light is right. That's the way it's supposed to be.
Me: Who do you think the light is?
Grace: Jesus Christ. (Then Grace went on to say:) I've got to go the bathroom, about to die!
Me: (About half an hour had passed) Do you still see the light?

Grace: Yes

Me: What is it saying?

Grace: Come unto me, come unto me, come unto me you who are heavy laden, heavy laden.

During this discourse, I took Miss Grace's vital signs, and they were all stable, and oxygen saturation levels were normal. I was absolutely astonished at what I had witnessed and the conversation I had with her, as Miss Grace was never able to have conversations like this. This was more than a visioning experience. Visioning refers to a patient seeing someone from their past, loved ones who have gone on before them.

This was more like a practice run before departure with what she was saying and her hand gestures of pointing and almost trying to hold and embrace those she was seeing. She was in another realm that was not this physical earth.

Because I was ignorant of this phenomenon, I kept asking Miss Grace questions rather than encouraging her to go toward the light. I was so caught up in what was happening that I didn't even think to look if she was a DNR, and she wasn't. Thankfully, she didn't die that night!

The next day, her vitals were altered, and she was sent to the hospital to be treated for an infection. When she came back a few days later, she was bedbound and didn't get up anymore. She was not eating, only sipping fluid.

She died approximately three weeks after this spiritual realm event happened. I was stunned. Not often do people have such clear communication that they are willing or able to speak what they see in the spiritual world.

The staff was shaken as they couldn't believe what she was communicating. We talked about it for days after. It raised many questions about the whole process and intricacies when we start to detach from the physical shell of our human existence. It made me yearn for more information about the dying process. I wanted to help patients in every aspect, including the physical, emotional, and spiritual realms.

When I started to write this story, I was going from my memory of 28 years ago. Thankfully, I was re-organizing my office space and found the documentation buried in my early hospice years folder.

I'm glad I wrote this down when it happened because not once have I been privileged to experience a conversation like this in my Hospice years.

Thank you, Miss Grace, for enlightening someone who was too young to be *approved by the light.* Your words inspired my journey into the world of hospice!

DARKNESS

I have been debating heavily in my mind and heart whether or not I should write this story. The fact that it is such heavy contemplation expresses that I need to even though I don't want to. It is amazing how recollections can stay embedded deep in your mind with a haunting recall. I write this story for education and to describe what a horrible death can look like. This is a vivid memory 24 years later. It occurred during my first hospice employment as a case manager back east when I was 28 years old.

Elaine was diagnosed with NHL, non-Hodgkins lymphoma. She was in her early 50's. The oncologist had done everything, including multiple forms of chemotherapy, radiation, and experimental trials. When the referral came in, we were told this would be a challenging case as Elaine was incredibly angry. She told off her oncologist with fuming words and also directed her anger toward God, and abandoned her faith of many years with multiple expletives.

Her children were grown, and she lived with her husband in a beautiful grand home in a prestigious subdivision. I recalled walking into her home for the first time and admiring the beautiful décor and layout of her three-story home. Everything had an exact place to be. It was not an illusion of perfection; it was real. It was disturbing how perfect her surroundings were. I didn't understand the dynamics of this as the team was not made aware of the details of her history. Her stay on service was only a few weeks.

Elaine's pain was neuropathic in nature, and her primary pain management was delivered via a pain pump to her IV port access.

Dilaudid was the narcotic of choice at this time. This was in the year 2000. I was two years into case managing and learning every day.

I had only visited Elaine a couple of times when the call came in that she was in a tremendous pain crisis, which started in the early morning. I arrived to find her on the lower level of her home, where the once beautifully decorated room had been transformed into her room with all the equipment, including a hospital bed and supplies. Her pain pump had been set to 60 mg of Dilaudid per hour.

I called our medical director, and he gave me parameters for implementing the next few hours of titration. These adjustments did not help. Elaine continued to cry out in agony. I was alarmed by what I witnessed, so I asked my supervisor for help. She sent out a more seasoned nurse who worked in the hospital setting and did hospice on the side.

I was thankful when she arrived because dealing with Elaine's spouse was more of a challenge than what I had the maturity to handle. Allen, Elaine's husband, would state over and over again how the Oncologist promised him and Elaine, 'She would not die in pain.'

The Dilaudid was increased to 400 mg/hr. We called our medical director again. It took over an hour for a response. We told him what had played out over the past several hours, and he could hear her screaming in the background. I asked if she could go to the hospital and get a nerve block. The medical director agreed, and Allen agreed, so we called 911.

When the ambulance arrived, Allen indignantly changed his mind and shouted, "No! She would not go to the hospital to die there." I begged him to change his mind as it was clear the Dilaudid was not working, and she needed methods of pain control we couldn't provide in the home setting.

Allen was in so much torment as he had not been processing losing his wife. Allen wanted complete control, and as Elaine's POA and spouse, we had to abide by his wishes. We followed the doctor's orders and kept increasing the Dilaudid basal rate, which hit the 1000 mg/hr mark.

One hour after this titration, Elaine started to settle, only by a fraction. She didn't want to be in the hospital bed. She laid on the floor with blankets. Finally, her body rose upward, and she experienced seizure-like activity. Her face had a look of doom, and her color was grey/blue over her skin. Her eyes were dilated, and the look of anguish and fear as she took her last breath was a memory I wish I could erase. It was over.

This was the longest ten hours I had ever spent with a patient in such horrific pain. Elaine's pain was not just physical but also included the elements of emotional, mental, and spiritual anxiety. Her pain involved many processes and factors. Healthcare providers today refer to this as functional neurological symptoms disorder.[29]

This experience shook me so much that I couldn't stop crying for three days. I could not work. I had to take a few days off. I composed my thoughts and wrote out everything that transpired and how I felt different decisions could have been made. The medical director should have made a home visit to intervene. He had the ability to do so. I felt like my nursing cohort and I were abandoned by our team to deal with such a horrific dying experience.

This was a learning experience of monumental proportions, and we talked about this in detail at the following interdisciplinary group meeting and came up with a plan for if this ever occurred again.

Medications are only one part of the picture to help someone have a peaceful death. When issues go unresolved, and anger resides in one's heart, leaving this world peacefully is not possible. Life is taken from us, or we can *choose* to let it go. Righteous anger is a natural response to patient suffering. This is called 'normalization.' Normalizing anger can help patients embrace and move through the anger phase of the dying process.[30] Elaine and Allen did not process the anger phase of the dying process in the anticipatory grieving stage, and the outcome was very unfortunate.

---

[29] Cleveland Clinic, "Psychogenic Pain: What It Is, Symptoms & Treatment, "https://www.ncbi.nlm.nih.gov/pmc/articles/PMC181044/.

[30] PubMed Central, "The Angry Dying Patient," https://www.ncbi.nlm.nih.gov/pmc/articles/PMC4262557/.

> **Hospice Highlights**
>
> - Engage the Interdisciplinary Team immediately in a crisis.
> - Process with your team situations that could have better outcomes.

Source

29) Cleveland Clinic. "Psychogenic Pain: What It Is, Symptoms & Treatment."
30) PubMed Central. "The Angry Dying Patient." https://www.ncbi.nlm.nih.gov/pmc/articles/PMC4262557/.

LOVE IS BLUE

I was honored to see the following story unfold before my eyes. I came for my visit with John toward the last half of this dialogue. It is rare when patients are transitioning into the spiritual realm that they can talk so clearly and vividly. Kaye, John's daughter, wrote the following conversation with their pastor present.

"Although it was the most difficult thing I have ever done, I am very thankful that I was able to grant Dad's final wish to cross over from his own home and thank God for the strength to get through. During the early morning hours of his last day, Dad and I were alone. After a while, I decided to write down everything he said so that the rest of the family could read his words. I know that the best thing that came out of the day was the confirmation of our beliefs and the comfort of knowing that he was on his way to heaven and was already in the arms of Jesus."

John's statements are in italics.

God. (pointed straight up)
Always.
Heaven waits
Blue!
Love is blue.
Help me, Jesus!
Please, honey, tell me.
Help me, Jesus.
Who is that? (pointed to a spot behind me)
Help me, Lord (reached up with both arms)

Heaven, look at…would you show…so beautiful!
Baby.
Yes, yes, we are going.
Once the chosen.
Watch her now
Surprised how good this…that was the stars…where did it go?

Pastor: John, do you know who I am?

John: Yes

Pastor: Are you talking to the Lord?

John: Yes

Pastor: Praise the Lord

John: Praise the Lord

Pastor: Debby is praying for you, too.

John: I appreciate that.

Pastor: Are the comforting arms of Jesus around you now?

John: Yes

Pastor: I'm sorry you are having such a hard time.

John: Tough…between the two.

Pastor: Are you in a lot of pain?

John: Yes, help me, you sure can.

Pastor: Do you know me?

John: Yes

Pastor: We've known each other for a long time, read the scriptures, and we know Heaven's a wonderful place, and you are going there.

John: Yes, help me

Pastor: He is helping you; hold to his hand, never doubt.

John: Thank you Jesus

Pastor: At the cross, at the cross.

John: Help me.. tell him.. forever… in Heaven.. tell us.

Pastor: Are you talking to Jesus? Have you seen Jesus this morning?

John: Has he made a voice yet? Ready. I'll show you. Heart is right. (pointed straight up and then to his heart.)

Pastor: Your heart is right with the Lord

John: Yes. Know something… It's all right…I love you Jesus. Yes, it is….I'll say goodbye. Jesus, Savior…Love you Lord Jesus…He is my Savior. God be sure to love…Thank you…Hear me Lord…I Love the Lord.

Pastor: It's OK.
John: Yes
Pastor: The Lord is my Shepard
John: I'll meet you. How are the girls?
Pastor: Fine, they are fine.
John: Is that you? Heaven's not far…Who's that? Not alone… He is here. Yes…They'll be all right. Yes, Lord, I love you. Help me. Betty…Angels…Just a little bit…The Light…
Kaye: Just reach for it, Dad.
John: I already did.

"Most of what Dad said after this point was impossible to understand completely right up until he crossed over when we were all singing the hymn, How Great Thou Art. He joined in and very clearly sang along with us. He crossed over minutes after into perfect peace."

The recounting of this dialogue is so incredibly unique in the dying experience. Usually, oxygen levels are so low that patients cannot articulate words with such countenance. Even though John was receiving small amounts of pain medication during this process, it was interesting to note his words when he said "yes" to having pain. Sometimes, the "pain" experienced is in the spiritual realm when it is so hard to let go of everything we've ever known on this physical earth and leave the ones we hold so close to our hearts.

Seeing this beautiful expression from John impacted me greatly, as this was my first year as a hospice nurse back in 1999. I encouraged the family to keep writing down every word, and Kaye did exactly that. This would be a special treasure to pass on to the future generations that would follow, how her father transitioned to the realm where *Love is Blue*.

TRAVEL TALK

The following are brief snippets/stories of how patients talked with very specific verbiage before making their departures. This can happen a few days before death or even several weeks before dying. In terms of crossing over to the next realm, travel talk involves a mechanism of how to get there, clothes and items that are needed, forms of movement and action, and visible people instructing them it is time.

CHIEF

I had known Chief for many decades growing up on the mountain. He was a very strong-willed man, set in his ways, and a true pioneer. I was on call for a 72-hour weekend. The family had requested hospice help as he was in his last weeks, curled up in a fetal position on his couch.

After getting him secure in the hospital bed for comfort, I received a call from his wife. She couldn't get him comfortable with the medications, so I visited. Chief was in transition when I arrived. His oxygen levels were dropping, and he was very restless. He kept uttering soft words that I couldn't understand as he was so weak.

Finally, he slowed his speech enough for me to hear what he was saying, *"How-do-I-get-out-my-body?"* He repeated this several times and looked me straight in the eye, demanding an answer. I encouraged him to go toward the light and let go of his earthly body. God was waiting for him and to reach for Him.

I knew he was a man of faith, so I prayed with him as best I knew how to deal with the feelings I anticipated he might be experiencing since I knew his history. Chief acknowledged the prayer and gave me a look that he understood. After a few more rounds of medications, he became calm and took his last breaths. I was thankful I could be there for his crossing over and with his precious wife.

CLARA

Clara was a long-time nurse and loved by many. She spent her last weeks being cared for in a skilled facility. She was related to one of my co-workers who wanted to know when she would start to transition so the family could be there 24/7. Clara's vital signs were stable, but the oxygen levels were slowly trending down.

Upon my arrival, I gently woke Clara to assess her pain levels. She quickly responded with determination in her speech, *"It's time to dance. I need to dance, go!"* She said this multiple times with her eyes closed. I knew her transition was starting. I informed the staff nurses, and educated them, as they weren't familiar with these peculiarities.

As I had brought her back to the present physical realm with conversation, anxiety, and pain started to escalate, so a schedule was written for symptom management with morphine for the shortness of breath and Ativan for anxiety. My next stop was to the office to inform my co-worker that it was time to gather the family. As Clara was telling us, it was time to dance. Clara passed peacefully one day later.

BETHANY

Bethany had just arrived at her beautiful home on the lake via ambulance from the hospital. It was late in the day, and she was content to be in her own surroundings again. It was summer, and temperatures in Alaska were around 50 to 60 degrees on average. This day was unusually warm for the land of the midnight sun in the 70s. The temperature in the house was quite warm, and the fans were on.

As I was going through the admission paperwork with the family, Bethany began asking for her winter coat, boots, and purse. She kept saying she needed these things now and wanted them on. The family kept re-directing her and telling her it was summer and she didn't need those things.

We quickly finished signing the papers, and I went straight to the Blue Book and began teaching them about the dying process. Even though her vital signs were stable and her passing did not look imminent, Bethany was travel-talking. She died two days later, surrounded by her family, with her purse on her bed, boots on the floor, and coat at the foot of the bed.

DUTCH

Dutch was on service for hemorrhagic stroke. He was the sweetest man. Mild anxiety was his most prominent symptom. His memory was short-term, and every visit felt like Groundhog Day. When I left that morning after my visit, I talked with his daughter about his care plan for the upcoming months. Utilizing agency help 24/7 was draining his bank account quickly. She started the process of investigating ALFs.

In the stand-up report the next morning, I was in absolute shock when I heard the news he had passed that night suddenly. Dutch had told his caregiver around midnight that he was ready to go home! The caregiver replied, "Dutch, you are in your own home right now." He said, "No, my heavenly home." He called his wife's name, Delores, and pointed at the door. He said, "She's standing right there by the door and calling me home!" The next second, Dutch took his last breath and died. Just like that!

Lisa

Lisa was six years old and my first pediatric patient in the early years of my career. Pediatrics hospice is a specialty all its own. I remember the challenges of working with Lisa as her parents wanted to do many interventions to keep her going. I can't imagine the pain and sorrow of slowly losing your child to cancer.

One visit, I was granted some rare time alone with Lisa as her mom was busy working in another room. Lisa opened up quickly and told me that her grandmother had been visiting her lately. She was so excited she wanted to tell someone. She told me she didn't think her parents would understand.

She would see her in the upper right corner of the room. Lisa said Grandma would stretch out her arms and tell her she could come home with her now. She explained, "She just keeps calling me and wanting me to go with her."

I encouraged Lisa to go when she was ready, and when she felt it was okay, for her to say goodbye to her mom and dad. Lisa's parents revoked hospice two days later, went to the hospital, and had a gastrostomy tube placed to feed her. They did not want to let their baby girl go.

She died three weeks later in that same hospital. It was not a peaceful death as they refused to stop the tube feedings, and she filled up with fluids in her lungs and throughout her body.

It is a privilege of information when patients give you hints about travel talk. It truly helps their loved ones prepare for the impending journey and enables them to come to the bedside and hold vigil if desired. Timing is unknown to the exact moment when the spirit will leave the body; therefore, it is imperative to pay special attention to how your patients communicate on this topic.

Do not dismiss these adjectives and verbs as 'talking out of their head or not making any sense.' These words paint an important picture in their transition. Their words are real and should be taken seriously.

When we die, we are getting ready to do something that we have never done before. Where is the confidence in this? We have never been taught how to separate from our bodies. But you, as the hospice nurse or family member can exhort, encourage, teach, and hold presence with your patient to help their body relax.

If you think of an automobile, one must turn the key off to shut the engine down. When the driving mechanism (the body) is turned off, the spirit can then leave its structure in the physical body. Tuning in to *travel talk* and responding in a positive and affirming manner to help the patient release is significant in aiding them in turning the key off.

Hospice Highlights

- Travel talk involves a mechanism for travel, movements or actions, clothing and personal items, and people giving instructions.
- Pay attention! Sometimes, the words are subtle and other times very bold.
- Affirm the dialogue taking place and place items next to the patient needed for travel as an affirmation.

BOUNDARIES

So, let's talk about boundaries. Yes, it's important to establish healthy boundaries to deliver quality care to your patients and to protect yourself emotionally. However, there seems to be one area where I seem to blow it, which is with the canines!

They are the innocent ones left behind after their loved ones have nurtured, cared for them, and given them their home. I am sure they feel abandoned and heartbroken when their person leaves this earth. I believe animals know what is happening to their human. They can smell the hormonal changes occurring as death approaches.

I've seen pets behave in various extremes. Sometimes, they want to be as close as possible, under or by the bed or lying in the bed with them at their feet. Other times, they distance themselves as they anticipate grieving.

When all is said and done, it is heartbreaking to see families negotiate to see who will feel the most obligation to take them in. When options have run out, I jump in from time to time. I do try to ration how often I can do this, though, as my daughter's house is now full of several rescues. Her heart is bigger than mine.

My latest gotcha dog is Sammy. He is eight years old, and he is all mine. His acquisition occurred a few days before Christmas. How could I let this precious dog go to the animal shelter after his owner had to go to the hospital and then to a facility for his remaining days since he lived alone and had no caretaker? I told Jake I would keep him until I could find him a good home.

I don't understand how he got my attention. He absolutely did not fit the profile! The first couple of times that I was around Sammy, he really didn't like me. He growled at me and stayed very close, guarding Jake fiercely. He was emitting endless hair everywhere he walked. He had not been groomed for over a year, if not longer.

It must have had something to do with those pale blue eyes, drawing me gently in. I am not one to be drawn to dogs that shed, that is for sure. I didn't know how severe the shedding would be since he was a mixed breed.

I was concerned because I tend to be a little allergic. What was I getting myself into? Was the holiday season mixed with the darkness outside, causing me to make a rash decision? Possibly...

As Jake went to the hospital to get his symptoms under better control, I took Sammy to Bella's house for a bath to get rid of the smoke smell. A long overdue grooming session was necessary. He was a bit traumatized by all the emotions of leaving his person and enduring a very thorough spa day that lasted several hours. To this day, Bella is not his favorite. In Sammy's defense, she does like to tease him like a little brother!

I brought him home that night and kept him on a leash as he went to every corner of the house, smelling all the boundaries. He quickly settled in and started following me like a service dog everywhere I went. I was only intending to foster him for a while. I did not plan to bond with Sammy. I couldn't help it; I fell for those sweet blue eyes and that elegant tuxedo coat appearance. I guess God knew I needed a gentle companion who would be devoted to me.

He loves to snuggle, unlike any other dog I've ever owned. Jake warned me that he likes to sleep in the bed, and this is the only place he would sleep. He has steps to help him up to his side of the bed and his multiple blankets. He is my partner on daily walks morning and night and demands the routine.

Jake told me he was a blend of Boston terrier and Pitbull. After doing the genetic test, it revealed husky and lab as well as a touch of bulldog. Being a short-haired dog, he doesn't shed much. I endure the occasional sneezes and stay on top of his brushing. He's worth it.

It may be a boundary broken, but one that brings joy to my heart every day. I will keep Sammy during his Hospice years until he crosses the rainbow bridge.

AURORA

I carry myself upon the currents of an endless western shore
From timeless night to sleepless day, I say a whisper of folklore
Recapture to create hidden inner sanctum
One I wish could stay peaceful and quiet as once I had clasped them
The sparkles of this sapphire night fade as currents travel
From fallen sun to frontier morn
Twill tell the story years of early born

I wrote this poem 33 years ago, on a flight home for Christmas break from college. While flying across the country heading back to the great white north, we encountered strong weather patterns of snow. As we crossed into Alaskan air space, the snow ceased, and the amazing Aurora appeared.

Flying through the brilliant colors of multiple shades of green and sapphire felt mystical and spiritual together. I felt like the whole world lay ahead of me with so many hopes and dreams that were yet to be fulfilled. At this time, I had no idea that nursing was the field I would be entering, let alone the specialty of hospice and end-of-life care.

I often recall this poem when I see Aurora. It prompts me to think of my patients and what they are seeing and experiencing in the spiritual realm in the days prior to their crossing over. What are their senses engaging with? I can only wonder.

On a Friday night in March, after an intense week of work, the alerts were coming out that the Aurora would soon be visible and strong that night. (March and October are the two most prominent months for Aurora in Alaska). My daughter, Bella, who was 19 at the time and still living at home, drug my exhausted body out of bed at 11 pm. On a hunt we went, in the cold temperatures of negative five degrees Fahrenheit, to chase the spectacular colors.

She was so excited to get going, that neither one of us dressed properly for the frigid temperatures. Coats and hats were put on, while gloves were forgotten. We did remember our iPhone to capture pictures.

We started on the back roads with wide open fields to watch the dance begin. Our eyes observed the patterns of the purple, pink, and red waves of brilliance. The waves appeared like angels' wings moving quickly as if they were telling a story. They acquired new shapes and forms during their eloquent dance.

Standing right below the center of this dance, we heard a crackling noise with a static background. It was truly unbelievable. I had no idea that the Aurora could emit a frequency. After all my years of living in Alaska, it blew my mind that there could be something audible that could accompany this light show. It felt like we were in the presence of something divine. I imagined maybe this is what it is like when people cross over into the next realm. The unimaginable beauty of color in terms we can't even comprehend, along with a frequency of language that we have yet to be able to articulate.

Over the next hour, we drove around the neighborhood, finding areas with fewer outdoor lights so the Aurora would be more visible from our vantage point. We kept going back inside the warm car with heat blasting to thaw our fingers out, then went back to the elements to take more pictures.

What an invigorating way to end a busy work week. Alaska can speak deep into your soul through its miraculous displays of nature. We must make the time to participate, even at midnight!

Conclusion

It has been quite a journey writing this book over the course of two and a half years. It is hard to express what it's like to be on the receiving end of inspiration and flow and then experience times having to push through to find fruition. The concept of perseverance and patience have taken on new meaning in my heart and life. I hope these stories from people who were very dear to me will find a place in your heart as you walk through the journey of being a hospice nurse or a caregiver to your family member.

There are so many topics that can be written about in the world of hospice. My wish is that these chronicles provide a deeper understanding of disease process, pain and symptom management, and the grieving process in the home setting, as it can be different than the hospital.

Walking alongside patients through the physical, spiritual, mental, and emotional realms is a beautiful privilege. I couldn't ask for a more fulfilling job as a nurse, being a part of an amazing hospice team to deliver quality care to patients. It is an honor to meet people where they are at while they journey through the dying process, being able to bestow love, kindness, and compassion as they write their final life chapter and cross into the next realm where love is blue.

Resource Page

1) A Tale of Three Men: Bargaining

Medicare. "Medicare-Certified 4 Levels of Hospice Care." *Medicare.gov.* https://www.medicare.gov/coverage/hospice-care

2) Humor

National Hospice and Palliative Care Organization. "CHC Compliance Guide." *National Hospice and Palliative Care Organization.* https://www.nhpco.org/wp-content/uploads/CHC_Compliance_guide.pdf.

3) I will Decide

Macy Catheter. "Macy Catheter." *Macy Catheter.* https://www.macycatheter.com/.

4) Life Review

"The Five Stages of Life Review." *Verywell Health.* https://verywellhealth.com/the-five-stages-of-life-review-1132503.

www.ingramcontent.com/pod-product-compliance
Lightning Source LLC
LaVergne TN
LVHW040858131224
799040LV00008B/179